Could it be You?

Overcoming dyslexia, dyspraxia, ADHD, OCD, Tourette's syndrome, autism and Asperger's syndrome in adults

DR ROBIN PAUC

WITH CARINA NORRIS

First published in Great Britain in 2008 by
Virgin Books Ltd
Thames Wharf Studios
Rainville Road
London
W6 9HA

A catalogue record for this book is available from the British Library.

ISBN 978 0 7535 1339 2

The Random House Group Limited supports The Forest Stewardship Council [FSC], the leading international forest certification organisation. All our titles that are printed on Greenpeace approved FSC certified paper carry the FSC logo.
Our paper procurement policy can be found at
www.rbooks.co.uk/environment

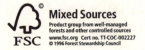

Mixed Sources
Product group from well-managed forests and other controlled sources
www.fsc.org Cert no. TT-COC-002227
© 1996 Forest Stewardship Council
FSC

Typeset by Phoenix Photosetting, Chatham, Kent
Printed and bound in the UK by
CPI Mackays, Chatham ME5 8TD

CONTENTS

ABOUT THE AUTHORS

Robin Pauc DC DACNB FCC

Robin Pauc graduated from the Anglo-European College of Chiropractic in 1974. He studied neurology at postgraduate level in the Netherlands before qualifying in the USA. He was later awarded a professorship at the prestigious Carrick Institute at Cape Canaveral. He has lectured and taught clinical neurology internationally and has written several books including the bestselling *Is That My Child? (UK)/The Learning Disability Myth (USA)* and *The Brain Food Plan* with Carina Norris. He is currently the director of the Tinsley House Clinic UK.

Carina Norris MSc (Dist), RNutr

Nutrition consultant, author and journalist Carina Norris studied biology followed by Public Health Nutrition. She was the nutritionist for Channel 4's *Turn Back Your Body Clock*, and has written several books on health and nutrition, including *You Are What You Eat: The Meal Planner That Will Change Your Life*, *Turn Back Your Body Clock*, *You Are What You Eat: Live Well, Live Long*, and co-authored Lorraine Kelly's *Junk-Free Children's Eating Plan*. Carina is now working on a PhD on children's nutrient intake. She has a passion to spread the word on healthy 21st-century living and help people dejunk their diets – the fun way.

1

INTRODUCTION TO DEVELOPMENTAL DELAY

Many people have tried unsuccessfully to find a treatment for learning and behavioural difficulties. At Tinsley House Clinic we now believe that the reason an effective solution has been elusive is that everyone has been looking in the wrong place.

The problem is the way learning and behavioural difficulties are classified and labelled: as conditions including dyslexia, dyspraxia, attention deficit hyperactivity disorder (ADHD), attention deficit disorder (ADD), obsessive-compulsive disorder (OCD), autism and Tourette's.

We need to redefine the problem. It is my belief that *all* of the conditions named above are really *symptoms* rather than *conditions*, and they are, in fact, symptoms of a wider underlying problem in the way that certain brain cells develop. To be precise, it is a developmental delay concerning certain brain cells, a concept we will return to again and again.

I believe that the misleading labels – dyslexia, dyspraxia, ADHD and the like – should be replaced by the general term Developmental Delay.

BORN TOO SOON

In order to understand the new ways in which learning/behavioural problems can be treated, not only in children but adults as well, it is essential to know how the human brain functions – how it has developed and evolved and how this can potentially impact upon our personal development. We must therefore look at not only that which is generally known about how the brain develops, but also a gaping hole in our knowledge that to date has led to the misdiagnosis of learning disabilities and has held back appropriate effective treatment.

All human babies are born prematurely. That may sound like a bold statement but it's perfectly true. Although every other organ of the body is perfectly formed at birth (or very shortly afterwards), only needing to grow, the human brain is still in an embryonic state and continues to grow rapidly.

Why is this? Over evolutionary time, the human brain has evolved to be bigger, and this obviously means the skull needs to be bigger too. This bigger skull encasing the bigger brain has created a problem – namely, the skull has become too big to easily pass through the bony rim of the birth canal.

Birthing strategies

Mother Nature has come up with various strategies to get round this but, as you will see, these are not always perfect solutions.

Marsupials (kangaroos and the like) get round the problem by giving birth to a tiny joey that, with a little help from Mum, crawls up to the pouch (second womb) and there, in this highly elastic sac, increases in size some 2,000 times.

Dolphins have dispensed with the pelvis, an option not open to landlubbers, so that a baby dolphin can continue to grow until it is ready to join Mum and Dad without the necessity of passing through the unforgiving bony ring of the pelvis.

Neanderthal man – or rather woman – attempted to get around the problem by developing a much bigger pelvis. However, a much bigger foetus requires an enormous amount of food and from a mechanical perspective is extremely difficult to keep in place, particularly as a biped (two-legged animal). Hence, Neanderthal woman became extinct and only her legacy lives on – 'Does my bum look big in this?'

Modern man (and, to a lesser extent, the great apes) has attempted to get around the problem by the female giving birth prematurely. That is, she gives birth at a stage when the foetus is undeveloped enough to still pass through the birth canal. This is a good strategy, apart from the fact that not all babies can pass through the birth canal with ease (they have a 'difficult' birth), and once born the relatively undeveloped baby requires constant care over a very long period of nurturing.

This extended period of nurturing has been called juvenilisation.

- Juvenilisation is the baby's extended dependency on its mother
- The human brain is still embryonic in form at birth
- It continues to grow rapidly long after birth
- During this time the brain must not only develop/mature but also learn
- The human brain has a great capacity to learn
- During the period of juvenilisation the brain is most susceptible to environmental influences

VON ECONOMO CELLS

In order to understand learning disabilities, we need to introduce a very special type of cell.

Von Economo cells were discovered in the 1920s by Constantin von Economo. For various reasons, their importance remained ignored for many years, and it is only recently that their significance has been appreciated.

These cells appear to play an important role in:

- The development of intelligent behaviour
- Responding to changing conditions/situations
- Dealing with conflicting thoughts
- The recognition of errors and avoidance of errors
- Deciding to act
- Increased activity associated with love/anger/lust
- Control of blood pressure, heart rate, breathing and digestion

Second-generation cells

To anyone interested in neuroscience the 'rediscovery' of von Economo cells was exciting enough, but what was to follow was truly mind-blowing. Although around 6 per cent of von Economo cells are present at birth, the vast majority do not start to develop until around four months later. That is, they form part of a **second generation** of brain cells.

It is generally accepted that all human organs are complete at birth with the exception of the brain, which continues to grow rapidly, but what no one had realised was that following birth completely new cell types start to form.

The special cells

So, what is so special about von Economo cells?

- They are only found in two small areas of the brain
- They are only found in the brains of humans, the great apes and whales
- In humans (and only in humans) they develop around four months after birth

Why is this significant? These cells are found in the very front of the brain – the prefrontal cortex – which until fairly recently was known as 'the silent area', simply because no one knew what it did. Now we know differently and can say that many of the functions of this region are what makes us what we are as humans and is the home of decision-making.

There are considerably more von Economo cells on the right side of the brain than on the left. This is important because the left side of the brain is traditionally thought of as being the home of language (in most people) and lots of other clever things, while the right side of the brain was thought to be a little more primitive – and yet this is where we find far more of these rather unique brain cells.

The 'more primitive' right side of the brain is involved in approach/withdrawal behaviour. That is, in every new situation the right side of your brain has to evaluate the situation and decide if it is safe to stay where you are or you should try to get away. If you decide that it is indeed safe to stay in this new environment, then the left side of your brain will take over and examine the details of this new environment. In children, if the right side of the brain is not developing (maturing) as quickly as it should, then the child will tend to avoid new situations and will prefer more familiar places and routine. In adults, when we are overtired or stressed we too prefer to be alone and avoid further stressful situations.

View of inner surface of the brain

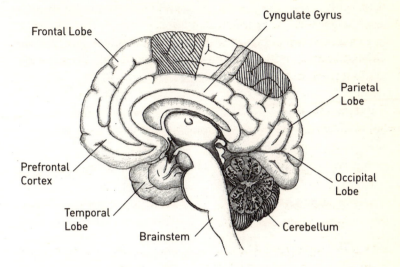

WALKING ON TWO LEGS

Something that is very unusual about us humans is that we are bipeds. In other words, when we are not sitting on our backsides we amble about on our hind legs. Apart from birds, we are the only animals on the planet to do this. It's true that apes, monkeys, rodents and marsupials *can* do this but they only walk upright when they want to, whereas we humans have to (unless we want to look incredibly stupid).

Being a biped has certain advantages. It makes us taller, which also means potentially we can see further, but it also frees our hands to do with what we will.

Let's look at vision for a moment. Being taller means we can see over things and perhaps get a better view of what is going on around us – useful if you want to survive – but if we could also improve our vision the advantage would be even greater, and that is effectively what we have done. By bringing the eyes in closer together we have been able to achieve stereoscopic vision. That is, each eye has a slightly different view of the world, which the brain then processes and fuses together thus giving us such things as perspective (the appreciation of depth) and the ability to judge the speed of an approaching object. If you don't believe me, try closing one eye and look at an approaching vehicle – but whatever you do, do not rely upon your judgement or you could end up as a statistic.

However, being a biped also has certain disadvantages. Anyone who has suffered the misery of low-back pain will tell you that walking upright puts a lot of strain on the spine and can potentially lead to a lot of visits to the doctor.

Walking on two legs has also led to a reduction in the size of the pelvis and hence the bony birth canal, which has in turn provided a limit to the size of skull that can pass through it – which itself determines the maximum size a baby's brain can be at birth.

The eyes have it

Moving the eyes in closer together also means that our noses have to be small enough to fit in between them, and this has led to certain changes within the brain. Now it would appear that the smell-related (and digestive) functions of two regions of the front of the brain have been taken over during our fairly recent evolutionary history to become involved in cognition – in other words, thinking. And what's truly astounding about this is that very few people on the planet, including most neuroscientists, know it. Hence, I have called these areas of the brain lying on the medial wall the **'dark side'** of the brain.

I really do believe that the areas of the brain we are going to be considering in this book have been not only misunderstood in the past but, because of this, have been relegated to a position of little importance compared with other regions of the brain's cortex.

Therefore, we must not only concentrate on redefining the importance of the right side of the brain but also highlight the functions of areas of the brain that lie hidden between its hemispheres.

Summing up

Before moving on perhaps we should have a little recap on what we have said so far and then look at the possible problems this might cause in terms of brain development and, in particular, learning disorders.

1) The brains of the great apes, whales and humans contain unique brain cells not found in any other species.

2) In the great apes and humans they are found in only two distinct regions of the brain.
3) In humans these cells are bigger, we have more of them and they are concentrated in the right side of the brain.
4) Only in humans do these cells develop after birth.
5) In humans they develop some four months after birth, which means their development can be hindered by any birth trauma.
6) Because we are born very prematurely we have an extended period of nurturing – juvenilisation – during which time the environment has the potential to have an impact on their development.
7) The human brain has increased in both size and complexity over the course of evolution.
8) The functions of the inner walls of the brain have changed with the development of the second-generation cells.

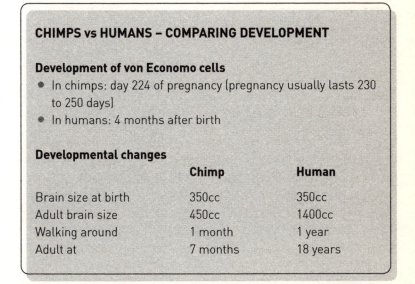

CHIMPS vs HUMANS – COMPARING DEVELOPMENT

Development of von Economo cells
- In chimps: day 224 of pregnancy (pregnancy usually lasts 230 to 250 days)
- In humans: 4 months after birth

Developmental changes

	Chimp	Human
Brain size at birth	350cc	350cc
Adult brain size	450cc	1400cc
Walking around	1 month	1 year
Adult at	7 months	18 years

Disorders Associated with Delayed Development of Second-generation Cells

Many conditions associated with the brain and behaviour involve these later-developing cells:

- Dyslexia
- Savant ability
- Autism
- Disturbances of thought
- Disturbances of language
- Withdrawal from social contact
- Schizophrenia
- Alzheimer's disease
- Attention deficit disorder (ADD)
- Learning/behavioural disorders
- Depression
- Obsessive-compulsive disorder (OCD)
- Phobic states
- Anxiety disorders

THE STRESSFUL EXPERIENCE OF BIRTH

If we return for a moment to the actual moment of birth, we have, as I mentioned earlier, the problem of the baby's head having to fit through the birth canal, and often it is a bit of a struggle to get it through. Sometimes, if a birthing problem is foreseen, an elective (chosen) Caesarean section can be performed, but often the baby just gets stuck and an emergency Caesarean has to take place or the baby has to have an assisted delivery with either ventouse suction or forceps. Foetal distress and assisted deliveries have been shown to significantly increase the probability that the child will go on to experience learning and/or behavioural problems. This really should not come as any great surprise, as all babies are effectively premature and some of their brain cells have yet to develop, let alone move off to that part of the brain where they are going to live and then hopefully function normally.

BPOPTOSIS

In 2004 the term bpoptosis was coined to describe the development, migration and making contact with other neurons of the second-generation neurons. Why bpoptosis? Well, it's a play on words, connected with an existing word, *apoptosis*. When the brain starts to form, a special tissue called neuroepithelium produces millions of brain cells. However, if these cells are to survive, once they have developed they must migrate and, once they have reached their final position, make contact with other neurons. Failure to do this equals certain death. The pruning of neurons, which varies considerably from individual to individual, is called apoptosis – programmed cell death. As no one in any textbook I have ever come across has ever mentioned the development of the second generation of brain cells, it seemed appropriate to coin a new term – bpoptosis – and create a little academic joke at the same time.

Bpoptosis: a term coined in 2004 to cover the window for the:
- Development
- Migration
- Making contact
of all second-generation neurons

The way the brain's second generation of neurons develop, move to their eventual destinations and make contact with other brain cells, and the impact this has had upon the dark side of the brain forms the foundation of a theory as to the cause and nature of learning and behavioural disabilities in children. However, as we will see, if left untreated these disabilities will not magically disappear when children reach puberty and become adults, but can blight an individual's entire life.

I am convinced that this does not have to happen and that with the right treatment all learning and behavioural problems can be addressed and treated successfully.

To see how this can and does happen we must look at how learning/behavioural disabilities have been looked at historically and hopefully learn from the errors of the past, so we can take a new look at the current situation.

In Summary

- Humans walk on their hind legs
- Walking upright restricts the size of the pelvis
- A bigger brain needs a bigger skull
- A large skull combined with a woman's small pelvis makes giving birth difficult
- All human babies are effectively born 'prematurely'
- The human brain is incomplete at birth
- A second generation of brain cells develops after birth
- Premature birthing means human babies need care for longer than other species of animal
- During this extended period of care the brain is most vulnerable

2

THE HISTORY OF LEARNING DISABILITIES – DYSLEXIA/ DYSPRAXIA

WHAT IS DYSLEXIA?

The word 'dyslexia' comes from the Greek and means 'difficulty with words'.

The British Dyslexia Association definition

Dyslexia is a specific learning difficulty which is neurobiological in origin [coming from the brain] *and persists across the lifespan.*

It is characterised by difficulties with phonological processing [processing the sounds in language], rapid naming, working memory, processing speed and the automatic development of skills that are unexpected in relation to an individual's other cognitive abilities [the abilities to think and know].

These processing difficulties can undermine the acquisition of literacy and numeracy skills, as well as musical notation, and have an effect on verbal communication, organisation and adaptation to change.

Put into plain English, dyslexia is a problem with not just reading but also how you deal with words, sentences and paragraphs in your head.

Potentially it can impair the ability to use letters, numbers and musical notes in a meaningful way. It is due to a problem in the brain and by this definition is incurable.

However, it may well be that it is not just brain processing that is the problem, as 57 per cent of children with learning disabilities attending a specialist clinic could not bring their eyes in towards their nose, to focus on an object, in a so-called convergence test. This has great implications for learning to read. Although it is perfectly possible to read with one eye, learning to read well does require the eyes to come in towards the nose before tracking the words across the page.

An amazing thing about people suffering from dyslexia is that the vast majority of them don't know it. A great many people who struggled to learn to read during childhood, and who now read slowly and dread having to fill out forms, may well have **secondary** dyslexia. That is, without realising it they may struggle to bring their eyes in towards the nose and then make both of their eyes track together across the page. In the clinic we can see and measure this problem using a computer-generated test, but at home you can get a very good idea if this problem exists with nothing more sophisticated than a pencil (see box on page 13).

Using Computers to Help Dyslexia

Convergence failure – secondary dyslexia
I do a simple convergence-failure test in the clinic and if I think there is a problem I use a computer-generated test to measure any problem accurately. The computer produces a 3-D picture that moves, making the eyes adjust the degree of convergence necessary to see the image. Another computer program then enables me to see if the patient's eyes are tracking – moving across the page together. The patient wears special goggles with built-in sensors to detect eye movements. The goggles are connected to a computer and the software superimposes the patient's eye movements over a passage of text that they read to themselves.

If I find there is a problem I use another computer program which the patient can take home with them and load on to their computer. On a daily basis the patient sits in front of the computer and completes a set of eye exercises. Depending on the results the computer decides when to make the various exercises more challenging. When the patient has reached a certain level the program tells the patient to contact the clinic, where (via the internet) their performance has been monitored. I can then switch the program to manual mode and tell the patient what to do next. Often it is necessary to continue using one part of the program to perfect one particular eye movement.

Does it work? In a trial conducted at a clinic, albeit using children, the program was 94.7 per cent effective.

THE DIY CONVERGENCE TEST

Have someone sit in front of you holding a pencil about 16 inches (40cm) from your nose. Stare at the end of the pencil while the pencil is brought in slowly towards your nose. The person sitting opposite you looks at the bridge of your nose and watches to see how your eyes move in towards your nose. The dominant eye – often the right – should move first but then the non-dominant eye should catch up and move in. Repeat this test at least three times.

Results

If both eyes move in and remain looking at the pencil, this is the normal response.

Alternatively, the following may happen:

- One eye – often the left – is slow to move in and struggles to stay on target.
- One eye – usually the left – starts to move in and then fails.

If one eye cannot hold fixation on the target, this is convergence failure.

What Causes Dyslexia?

Dyslexia Never Occurs Alone

Dyslexia is not a condition but a symptom, and a symptom that *always* occurs mixed with other symptoms – and all of them caused by developmental delay. So, if you have dyslexia the chances are you also have a little dyspraxia – you are a bit clumsy. You may also have aspects of attention deficit disorder – you lack concentration at times and are easily distracted.

Dyslexia tends to run in families, which suggests that it has a genetic basis. Over 70 per cent of the parents of children seen at the Tinsley House Clinic admit to having experienced learning or behavioural problems themselves. On the basis of my own research it appears that if there is a learning disability on the mother's side of the family there is a 30 per cent chance that one or more of her children may have a learning disability. If the problem is on the father's side of the family the probability shoots up to more than 70 per cent.

DNA is not destiny

If indeed dyslexia is genetic in origin (and to date a dyslexia gene has yet to be found) then it is not the end of the world. We now know that our genes are controlled by what is known as the epigenome – a set of protein switches. In a dramatic experiment using agouti mice it was shown that DNA is not destiny – diet can change the way genes express themselves. Agouti mice are large, round, yellow mice that as a rule die from cancer and/or diabetes. By changing their diet and notably adding a B-vitamin called folic acid, it was possible to change the genetic outcome in not only the offspring of the mice in the experiment but also that of their grandchildren. Remarkably, the baby mice were small, brown and did not die inevitably from cancer or diabetes, and nor did their offspring.

Stop searching for a dyslexia gene!

For years scientists have searched for a dyslexia gene or genes, but personally I think they will never succeed. Why? Because I believe that if they're interested in dyslexia, they need to be looking at the genes that control what is called morphogenesis. That is, the developing body and brain have to have a control system to set the timing for development – what to grow and when.

In the last few years it has been discovered that at around four months after birth a second generation of brain cells starts to develop (see Chapter 1). It is these brain cells, which are found predominantly on the right side of the brain, that give us the ability to carry out so many of the things that make us human. And this is where the importance of the morphogenesis genes comes in – they provide the instruction for these cells to start to develop and move off to where in the brain they eventually need to be.

Over the years scientists have come up with all sorts of reasons as to why people go on to develop such things as autism or dyslexia and one common factor keeps cropping up, namely stress. Not stress as in 'I am having a really bad hair day', but stresses on the body such as viral infections or rapidly fluctuating hormone levels. My own research has shown that foetal distress and/or birth interventions – ventouse delivery, etc. – increase the likelihood that a child will go on to suffer developmental delay (the various combinations of dyslexia, dyspraxia, ADD, etc.).

The discovery of the epigenome (those 'gene switches') and the amazing outcome of changing the diet of agouti mice have really given us all something to think about. Could biological stress during pregnancy, foetal distress, a difficult birth or even food additives eaten by the pregnant mother trip the switch and slow down or stop the development of the second-generation brain cells?

PRIMARY DYSLEXIA

So far we have considered the very real but as yet generally unrecognised condition known as secondary dyslexia. That is, an inability for certain parts of the brain to make the eyes move in (converge) towards the nose during close vision. When you last had an eye test or when your child last had an eye test, did the optician test for convergence failure? The answer is probably not. If convergence testing was part of every eye test and every child was tested in primary school I am convinced that the number of people with 'dyslexia' would fall dramatically.

We must now ask ourselves, 'Is there such a thing as primary dyslexia?' Well, the first thing to realise is that dyslexia **does not exist** as a condition. Dyslexia is a symptom, a problem that some people have with reading, spelling, comprehension, etc., but a symptom that will always be found together with dyspraxia and ADD or any of the other learning/behavioural problems. My own research has shown this to be the case and the evidence that has accumulated from around the world is now very convincing. So if we have a collection of symptoms – caused by a developmental delay concerning certain brain cells – why is it happening, and happening at a rapidly increasing rate?

Two halves that make a whole

The human brain has two sides, called hemispheres, and each hemisphere is concerned with different functions. In most people the left hemisphere will deal with clever things like language while the right side of the brain will put the lilt into what it is we are saying, amongst other things.

The right side of the brain is the approach/withdrawal side of the brain – should I stay or should I go? – while the left side of the brain has the ability to look carefully at the situation you find yourself in if the right side decides it is OK to stay. Put simply, the left side of the brain is the more academic, intellectual side, while the right side has generally been thought of as the more basic, primitive side. Be that as it may, the two sides have to work in harmony if the whole thing is going to function properly.

Brains out of synch

Joining the two halves of the brain is a structure called the corpus callosum. A lot of time and energy has been put into studying the corpus callosum and scientists have noted endless variations in size and form.

They have also, very recently and following a huge amount of research around the world, put forward a fascinating theory as to the cause of learning/behavioural problems.

Put very simply, the theory is that the two sides of the brain are out of synch. Each side of the brain should oscillate at a certain frequency (40Hz), setting a time frame in which brain activities can take place. Very interestingly, it seems that in most cases of learning/behavioural disorders, the problem originates on the right side of the brain. Although various names have been given to the underlying problem, it is basically a matter of not enough connectivity. That is, the connections between the different areas of the right hemisphere are late developing, particularly the long-distance brain cells that connect the front and back of the brain.

The missing link

I believe that the missing link in this theory is the second generation of brain cells that develop four months after birth. Their structure, location and known connections make them prime suspects and provide a logical explanation for the symptom patterns of developmental delay.

WHERE DO SYMPTOMS COME FROM?

Right side of the brain – attention deficit disorder (ADD), attention deficit hyperactivity disorder (ADHD), obsessive-compulsive disorder (OCD), Tourette's syndrome and autism

Left side of the brain – Dyslexia

Diaschisis (one area changing the function of another) – Dyspraxia

WHAT IS DYSPRAXIA?

The word literally derives from two Greek words 'dys' (meaning ill or abnormal) and 'praxis' (meaning doing).

The Dyspraxia Foundation definition

> *Developmental dyspraxia is an impairment or immaturity of the organisation of movement. It is an immaturity in the way that the brain processes information, which results in messages not being properly or fully transmitted . . . Dyspraxia affects the planning of what to do and how to do it. It is associated with problems of perception, language and thought.*

Dyspraxia is therefore a medical term used to describe a situation in which a person finds difficulty in learning and/or performing basic and routine motor tasks (as opposed to something like tightrope walking, which a great many people might find challenging).

Mix and match

There is a huge and confusing array of terms used to describe dyspraxia – acquired dyspraxia, developmental dyspraxia, dyspraxia, verbal dyspraxia, oro-motor dyspraxia, eating dyspraxia, dressing dyspraxia, developmental co-ordination dyspraxia, etc. And I believe this is a very good clue that dyspraxia, like dyslexia, does not exist as a condition. That is, dyspraxia is a variable *symptom* and not a *condition*: it will appear in a form that is as unique as the individual.

The term comorbidity describes a situation in which two (or more) different conditions frequently occur together in the same individual. It is my belief, and that of an increasing number of other researchers, that developmental dyspraxia rarely if ever occurs in isolation but is perhaps the most common symptom that appears in comorbidity with the other so-called learning/behavioural disabilities: dyslexia, attention deficit disorder (ADD), attention deficit hyperactivity disorder (ADHD), obsessive-compulsive disorder (OCD), autistic traits and Tourette's syndrome.

Comorbidity within the group of learning/behavioural disabilities is not a new concept but to date has only been studied in isolation – dyslexia/dyspraxia, ADD/ADHD, ADHD/autism – therefore, as no one has looked at the bigger picture, I believe the true nature of the disabilities has been missed. The term developmental delay syndrome (DDS) is a more accurate description of the presenting condition.

The child is father to the man

Historically, problems associated with motor co-ordination/dyspraxia were considered to be of little significance as it was thought that following the transition from childhood into adulthood the condition would somehow miraculously disappear. Now we know that this is not the case and, untreated, the dyspraxia persists, often severely limiting the individual's progress in life both physically and mentally.

When we consider the number of children estimated to have aspects of developmental delay – up to 8 per cent for dyspraxia, 20 per cent for dyslexia, ADD, ADHD and 1 per cent for Tourette's syndrome of childhood – and transpose these figures to the adult population, the potential size of the problem becomes visible. Furthermore, when we consider the growing body of evidence that would suggest these conditions do not occur in isolation, the future looks bleak for those children who do not receive effective treatment.

THE HISTORY OF DYSPRAXIA

The first mention of dyspraxia in terms of a developmental motor disorder is attributed to Collier in the early 1900s. He used the term 'congenital maladroitness'. In 1937 Samuel Orton suggested that this abnormal clumsiness was 'one of the six most common developmental disorders, showing distinctive impairment of praxis' (normal motor control/movement).

Dr Sasson Gubbay is attributed with the introduction of the now very politically incorrect term, the 'Clumsy Child Syndrome', following the publication of *The Clumsy Child* in 1975. These children were described as being clumsy despite being of normal intelligence and when examined neurologically were found to be normal.

This last sentence is significant in that it provides a clue as to the functional division of the brain in terms of its development – the brain you are born with providing what we may term intelligence, while the second generation of neurons allowing this intelligence to become overt. It would also indicate that neurology has moved on since the 1970s and I would suggest that now these children would not be found to be neurologically sound following an appropriate examination.

A J Ayres provided a very interesting twist in the development of our understanding of developmental dyspraxia when in 1985 she suggested that it may be a disorder of sensory integration. This suggestion took the emphasis away from developmental dyspraxia as being purely a motor disorder and introduced the possible role of the sensory system in the aetiology (cause) of the disorder. The gist of her argument was that a deficiency in sensory integration (function) would produce both an inability to plan motor activity (movements) as well as to carry out the motor function smoothly, thus leading to dyspraxia.

Signs of the symptom

A number of signs of dyspraxia may be identified at various ages and certain factors commonly associated with developmental dyspraxia are of note. Below is a list of signs taken from current popular works on dyspraxia. Signs that may be associated with other learning/behavioural problems are marked with an asterisk or are highlighted in **bold**.

At birth:

- Foetal distress and/or assisted delivery including emergency Caesarean delivery.*

Pre-school:

- Delay in acquiring normal milestones, notably sitting unaided, crawling, walking and speech.*
- Delay in acquiring bladder control by day and (notably) at night.*
- Difficulties with balance in general.*
- Poor spatial awareness, with a tendency to bump into things and knock things over.
- Poor fine-motor skills.
- Inability to dress and undress or to sequence dressing.
- Inability to use a knife and fork, resorting in using the fingers or just being a messy eater.
- Often tired and irritable.*
- He/she may be heavy-handed/heavy-footed.
- May resort to walking on tiptoe, particularly when excited. **Commonly associated with autistic traits.**
- Will often be described as having poor muscle tone and/or hypermobile joints.
- May be awkward.
- May be sensitive to noisy environments and bright lights. **Commonly associated with autistic traits.**
- Difficulty standing still and waiting. Has to move. Commonly associated with **ADD/ADHD.**

In School:

- Difficulty in fastening clothes, e.g. doing up buttons and fastening shoelaces.
- Poor organisational skills.
- An inability to undertake activities without seeing their hands, e.g. combing hair and wiping bottom.
- Poor spatial awareness.
- Hates P.E.
- Numerous falls/accidents.
- Dislikes sports.
- Difficulty performing bilateral activities, e.g. using a knife and fork.
- Poor self-awareness.

- May struggle with knowing left and right. The child may be left-handed, right-footed and left-eye dominant.*
- Poor handwriting with reversals of letters and/or numbers. Often seen with **dyslexia.**
- Reading may be slow to develop or may deteriorate. Often seen with **dyslexia.**
- May exhibit poor spacing of written words.
- Difficulty with numbers.
- Cannot express themselves in writing. Often seen with **dyslexia.**
- Low self-esteem and/or anxiety.*
- Prefers routine.*
- Easily frustrated.*
- Easily distracted, with a tendency to daydream. Often associated with **ADD/ADHD.**
- Short attention span or difficulty in concentrating for more than a few minutes. Often associated with **ADD/ADHD.**
- May be a loner or conversely be disruptive in class. The class clown.*
- May have difficulty in copying text from a book or the board. Often seen with **dyslexia.**
- Speech can be flat, lacking lilt.
- Social skills may be poor and the child may make friendships with children younger than themselves or prefer adult company.*
- The child is more vulnerable to bullying.*
- Eating habits can be poor and the diet may be restricted or high in carbohydrates.*
- Poor pencil grip with hand/arm pain and often flexion (bending) of the wrist.
- Disorganisation may be evident, especially if the child is trying to understand a complex timetable, more subjects, a larger school and a variety of room locations.*
- May have difficulty in taking dictation or remembering detailed instructions.*
- Low self-esteem, anxiety and stress will affect how well they do academically.*
- Highly emotional/very changeable emotions.

As children, at home and in the school environment, we are protected, nurtured and can be given extra help if we are struggling. Once we leave home, get a job and have to earn a living things can be very different. Low self-esteem and poor social skills can make it difficult to establish meaningful relationships, and being accident-prone and a bit of a daydreamer may not exactly impress the boss. However, all is not lost. By understanding what dyspraxia is, and more importantly what it is not, help is at hand regardless of your age.

What causes dyspraxia?

Dyspraxia is a symptom that occurs in the company of other symptoms such as dyslexia and/or attention deficit disorder as part of a developmental delay. That is, in most cases the right side of the brain is slow to develop and therefore shows signs of this immaturity.

At the back of the brain just behind the brainstem lies the cerebellum (the so-called 'little brain'). It too has two hemispheres (sides), each of which works with the opposite cerebral (brain) hemisphere. If either the cerebral hemisphere or the cerebellar hemisphere on the opposite side is not working as it should do, then one hemisphere can throw the other out of synch.

Brains out of synch again

At the bottom of the brainstem, on either side, is a tiny area that produces a spontaneous pulse at 8–12Hz. This pulsation passes up to the opposite cerebellar hemisphere, which in turn passes on a pulsation to the top of the brainstem, which then passes the pulsation back down to where it started. These reverberating circuits set the timeframe for all movements of the body and therefore have to be the same on each side. When you carry out the tests below you may discover that you can't keep the two sides of your body moving in synch or that you miss the target – you show dysmetria.

These triangular circuits are also responsible for setting the timeframe for the cerebral hemispheres, even though they oscillate at 40Hz. If you think of an old-fashioned cine camera, each frame of the film captures a moment of time and so it is with the human brain. Everything that you think, feel or do must be within a timeframe – a frame of the film – or not only will your movements be out of synch but so will your thoughts – dysmetria of thought.

There are two other areas of the brain which we also need to consider before we look at just what can be done to help if you think you may have aspects of dyspraxia as part of a developmental delay syndrome. Not all of our visual system sees in the usual way we think of seeing. One particular area called the parietal cortex contains some special neurons called magnocellular cells (which simply means 'big cells'). Their job is to keep you informed of exactly what is going on around you and to detect movement. If for any reason this part of your visual system is under-functioning you will be less aware of your surroundings than you need to be.

On the inside wall of this same area is another region that can impact upon how you function in space. This area deals with the memory of not only where you are but where you are in relation to your immediate environment. Now if one or all of these areas is not working too well do you think you might bump into things, knock things over or frankly be a walking disaster area?

TESTING FOR DYSPRAXIA

TEST 1
Stand with your feet together, hands by your side with your eyes closed. Have a friend gently but firmly tap the upper arm just below shoulder level, firstly on the left then on the right. Repeat this two or three times. Note on which side it is hardest to keep your balance.

TEST 2
Sit with your arms outstretched and the index finger of each hand pointing directly at your partner's nose. With your eyes closed you must touch your nose and then point at your partner, firstly with the index finger of the right hand and then with the left. This should be repeated several times consecutively and must be done with the eyes closed. Note if one finger repeatedly misses the nose or if there is a slight hesitation before the finger touches the nose.

TEST 3
Stretch your arms out in front of you. With your eyes open turn your hands to the palm-up position and then rapidly alternate the

movement – palms down/palms up. Have a friend look for the hand that goes out of sync first or the elbow that bends.

TEST 4
Sit facing a friend with your elbows by your side and your fore-arms outstretched in front of you, palms upwards. Turn your hands palms down/up as rapidly as possible while keeping your elbows by your side. Note which hand goes out of synch first or which wrist bends, producing a waving movement.

The results
If two or more of the tests above were positive – you fell to the left, missed your nose with one finger and/or rapidly went out of synch when flipping your hands to and fro – then the chances are you are demonstrating signs of dyspraxia.

Treating dyspraxia

Treating dyspraxia in isolation is a total waste of time. However, treating dyspraxia as part of a developmental delay syndrome is not only achievable but also effective at any age. In the last five chapters of this book we will look at diet, supplementation and exercises, both specific and general, as well as computer-generated treatment programmes that have been used successfully to treat both children and adults. But before we do that we must look at the other symptoms that make up a developmental delay syndrome.

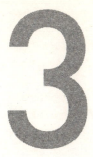

ATTENTION DEFICIT DISORDER

WHAT IS ADD/ADHD?

ADD/ADHD is now officially called attention deficit hyperactivity disorder, although most lay people, and even some professionals, still call it ADD or ADHD. The name has changed apparently as a result of scientific advances. This may be the case but it is my firm belief that it is because it is still considered as a condition in its own right that confusion reigns.

In an attempt to fit a square peg in a round hole it has not only been given a new name but is now divided into three subtypes, according to the main features associated with the disorder: **inattentiveness**, **impulsivity**, and **hyperactivity**.

> The three subtypes of ADHD are:
>
> * Predominantly combined type
> * Predominantly inattentive type
> * Predominantly hyperactive-impulsive type

How the classification is meant to work – and why it doesn't

These subtypes were created in the hope of taking into account the fact that some children have little or no trouble sitting still but may be inattentive and struggle to remain focused on the job in hand.

Others may be able to pay attention to a task (e.g. their PlayStation) providing they don't lose focus because of impulsive behaviour and/or a total inability to keep still. Not surprisingly, the most common subtype is the combined type, which contains elements of inattention, impulsivity and hyperactivity.

Not only does the presentation of these three elements vary but so do the other symptoms that it will be associated with. The presentation has to be as unique as the individual. However, the American Psychiatric Association publishes a great tome that contains all the diagnostic criteria for mental disorders from which all professionals have to work. So instead of looking at an individual we are meant to categorise everyone and squeeze round pegs into square holes.

But if you actually suffer from the symptoms described, the important thing to you is not how the condition should be classified, but what can be done about it, and this is what will be addressed in the rest of this chapter.

Diagnosing ADHD and ADD – The Eyes Have It

Thanks to a certain Professor Pavlidis, there is now an eye test that can be used to diagnose ADHD and dyslexia in preschool children. By checking four different eye movements for just two minutes it can be predicted with 93.1 per cent accuracy whether or not the child is likely to go on to develop a problem. At Tinsley House Clinic we use a computer program to do much the same thing and another computer-generated programme to correct any problems we find. To date we have found it to be extremely effective and the good news is that it works for adults too.

A HYPERACTIVE HISTORY

Attention deficit hyperactivity disorder was originally described by Dr Heinrich Hoffman in 1845, a physician with a penchant for writing medical books and poetry. One of his poems was entitled 'The Story of Fidgety Philip' and is a very accurate description of a child with ADHD.

Sir George F Still, a British doctor, produced a series of papers starting in 1902 in which he described a group of children who displayed impulsive behaviour. Although he called the impulsive behaviour a 'Defect of Moral Control' he did believe the underlying cause to be medical and not the result of poor parenting. Since that time the terminology has undergone considerable evolution, from post-encephalitic behaviour disorder through minimal brain dysfunction, hyper-kinetic reaction, attention deficit disorder, with and without hyperactivity, through to attention deficit hyperactivity disorder, the term in use today.

In 1937 Dr Charles Bradley introduced stimulant medication as a treatment for ADHD. Over the next several years he studied and published the results of medicating children exhibiting hyperactivity with Benzedrine and Dexedrine, describing how it affected their level of activity and school performance. Ritalin (methylphenidate) was first introduced in 1956 and remained the drug of choice until 1996 when Adderall was approved, to be followed in 1999 with Concerta, Strattera and others.

How Common Is ADD in Adults?

The exact prevalence of ADD in adults is unknown (in adulthood, the condition is usually referred to as attention deficit disorder, or ADD, rather than ADHD). Studies to date reveal that the condition, marked by inattentiveness, difficulty getting work done, and poor organisational skills, involves approximately 4 to 6 per cent of the US population, and it is likely to be similar in the UK. It can persist throughout a person's lifetime; approximately one-half to two-thirds of children with ADHD will continue to have significant problems with ADHD symptoms and behaviours as adults. This impacts not only on the life of the sufferer directly but also within the family, in the workplace and other social situations.

In one long-term follow-up study, up to 70 per cent of children with ADHD continued to have residual symptoms throughout adolescence and adulthood. These figures, based on a prevalence of 6 to 9 per cent in children, would predict a figure of 3 to 6 per cent in adults.

Attention deficit hyperactivity disorder in children is three times more common in boys than girls. Boys also have greater elements of hyperactivity, whereas girls often have the inattentive type. In adulthood, however, almost as many women have ADD as men.

CONTINUING POTENTIAL PROBLEMS OF ADULT ADHD AND ADD SUFFERERS

- Undereducated, low income, low status, little job satisfaction
- Antisocial and criminal behaviour, alcohol and drug abuse
- Mood swings, anxiety and depression
- Tic disorders
- Poor social skills, emotional problems, unstable relationships
- Road traffic accidents

Mapping the Mind

Much of what we know about brain function has come from doctors' detailed observations of their patients, as to their particular signs and symptoms. When the patients passed away the doctors could then note at postmortem the exact areas of the brain that had been damaged and gradually, over a period of time, they discovered which specific areas of the brain were responsible for which particular functions. Thus we now have a good idea of where a lot of brain functions and malfunctions are located, which means that to a certain extent they can be treated.

One particular medical anecdote throws a lot of light on the areas of the brain involved in ADHD. On 14 September 1848 in Cavendish, Vermont, USA, a foreman working on the railroad, Phineus Gage, was tamping gunpowder into a hole with a tamping rod. The story goes that he forgot to cover the gunpowder with sand and a spark from the tamping rod hitting a flint set the powder off, resulting in the rod being launched skyward. Unfortunately for Phineus his head was in the path of the projectile, which passed under his left cheekbone, through his left eye before entering his skull and finally exiting through the top of his head. Amazingly Phineus survived the accident and became something of a legend in medical history.

Apparently, before the accident he was an honest hard-working man employed by the railroad as a foreman with responsibility for rock blasting. After the accident Dr Harlow, his physician, reported that he had become a changed man. No longer a good timekeeper, he became foul-mouthed and was taken to drunkenness. He would create elaborate schemes that never came to anything, would lie and cheat and had no regard for social etiquette when it came to the fair sex.

One thing that everyone can agree upon is that the area of brain that lay just above Phineus's eyes was destroyed. A tamping rod over one inch in diameter and travelling at the speed of a rocket is going to cause a fair bit of damage, particularly when you consider that the brain has the consistency of cold porridge and the flat-ended rod would have been pushing ahead of it all the bone that stood in its way. This particular area of the brain is involved in what we might call the social graces, that is, behaviour considered appropriate for the society we live in. Little children, people who have had a little too much to drink and those suffering from dementia often demonstrate behaviour that is inappropriate. Little children do it because this area of the brain is underdeveloped, people who are intoxicated because the brain is effectively being poisoned, and those suffering the early signs of dementia because the von Economo cells we talked about earlier are the first to suffer with this condition.

Von Economo cells are found not only in the area that was destroyed in Phineus's accident, but also on the 'dark side' of the brain in the anterior cingulate area. When this area underfunctions it is very difficult to keep still, almost impossible to concentrate and everything that involves reading and maths seems harder than it should be. This is the underlying cause of ADHD, but it doesn't end here, as the areas that are in contact with this region will also be suffering. Hence it is unlikely that ADHD will occur alone, and far more likely that aspects of attention deficit will be found to occur with dyslexia, dyspraxia, etc.

Anyone who suffers from any form of developmental delay or anyone who lives with a sufferer will know that organisational skills and concepts of time are a major problem. Any parent will tell you that trying to tell a young child that you are in a hurry is a total waste of time, because young children have no concept of time whatsoever. In young children this is normal but as a child grows and develops, basic ideas of time should fall into place so that there comes a stage when we can actually have 'memories' of the future. That is, not only can we imagine what we are going to do on holiday but we can tell our friends all about it, even though it has not happened yet. If we can't do this as we grow up, major problems can occur when we leave home and either enter higher education or get our first job.

THE CAUSE AND EFFECT OF ADHD

The consensus of opinion is that ADHD is a neurobiological (brain-based) disorder. It has a strong genetic basis, and it has been suggested that ADHD is the most heritable of all mental disorders. Environmental factors such as drinking and smoking during pregnancy have been suggested as possible triggers. Certain areas of the brain of people with ADHD also work differently. Most significantly, they use glucose at a lower rate. Other studies have shown that the brain's anterior cingulated region underfunctions in people with ADHD and the situation worsens when they are mentally challenged or stressed.

Sugar junkies

What is so interesting about this reduced level of glucose metabolism is that a great many children and adults with ADHD are 'sugar addicts'. The vast majority of the patients I see that are fidgety to hyperactive live on a carbohydrate-laden diet that inevitably contains a huge array of additives and artificial sweeteners. It is as if they are constantly trying to top up their glucose levels but unfortunately fuelling their hyperactivity instead.

THE HADES DIET

- Breakfast – sugary cereals with added sugar with toast and jam. Squash.
- Snack – crisps, biscuits, cake and/or chocolate. Fizzy drink.
- Lunch – burger and chips or pizza or pasta. Fizzy drink.
- Snack – cake, biscuits and/or crisps. Squash.
- Dinner – pasta.
- Supper – sugary cereal or toast. Squash.

TREATMENT

The standard medical approach to treating ADHD in adults, when it is recognised, is to use medication and/or psychotherapy. Two types of medication are often considered: stimulants such as Ritalin and antidepressants.

Ritalin is a bit like Marmite – people, including experts, either love it or hate it. To the parents of a child that is out of control it can be a godsend, but to many others it is a controlled drug on a par with cocaine. Doctors who are in favour of using Ritalin will tell you that not only does it work but that the side effects are limited to such things as insomnia, loss of appetite and resultant weight loss in a few cases. The doctors who are not so much in favour of the drug paint a very different picture, which ranges from a worsening of the symptoms the drug is supposed to improve, to permanent abnormalities in the brain. For both children and adults, the one thing that is missing is believable research into the long-term effects of Ritalin and the other drugs used in the control of ADHD.

The rise of Ritalin

Originally, methylphenidate (Ritalin) was used to suppress the symptoms of ADHD (impulsiveness, lack of focus, hyperactivity) that effectively prevented the child from learning. As ADHD was thought to be a short-term condition that would resolve spontaneously with the onset of puberty, the suppression of symptoms would be of great benefit during school life. However, we now know this is not the case and that methylphenidate not only fails to effectively treat ADHD but also has potentially serious side effects.

General side effects of antidepressant medication

Some of the various side effects from the different antidepressants are:

- Dry mouth
- Urinary retention
- Blurred vision
- Constipation or diarrhoea
- Drowsiness, which can interfere with driving or operating machinery
- Disturbed sleep

- Weight gain
- Headache
- Nausea
- Stomach pain
- Inability to achieve an erection
- Inability to achieve an orgasm (men and women)
- Loss of libido
- Agitation/anxiety

NEUROTRANSMITTERS

Before going any further, we need a little more background on how the central nervous system works, and how the different parts of our body communicate with one another. Once you understand this, it will help you to see what is happening in the case of behavioural and learning problems, and how different treatments can help.

In a nutshell, in order to function, the brain and central nervous system has to transmit messages from cell to cell, between different regions of the brain, in order for you to think, make decisions, and take similar cognitive actions. Your nervous system also transmits messages from the brain, via the rest of the nervous system, to your muscles – this is what enables you to move various parts of your body. On top of this, there are also the unconscious movements and functions your nervous system co-ordinates without you needing to think about them – functions such as breathing, and moving your food along your digestive system. This is controlled by the so-called 'autonomic' part of the nervous system.

The nervous system's function is all about communication, and this is where neurotransmitters come in – they transmit messages from one nerve cell to another.

The cells in the nervous system aren't physically 'joined' – they are separated by tiny gaps called synapses, and messages have to 'jump' across these gaps. These jumps are performed by neurotransmitters. Cell number one releases a neurotransmitter, which passes across the synapse, and is then taken up by special receptors on the next cell along, enabling it to receive the 'message'. This cell, in turn, can pass the message on to cells that it is adjacent to, by releasing its own neurotransmitters for them to receive. In this way, chemical messages are transmitted around the body.

Three more words you need to learn in order to understand ADD and ADHD in particular.

Endorphin

It has also been said that high brain-sugar levels can alter the way that certain receptors work in the brain. A receptor is a site on a brain cell where it receives a specific chemical messenger called a neurotransmitter. One such transmitter is called an endorphin. It is the brain's natural painkiller and once released it gives you a feeling of euphoria – a high. If for any reason you are not producing enough endorphin your body will try to make up for it by producing more endorphin receptors, all the better to pick up the little endorphin that is available.

Serotonin

This is another neurotransmitter, and low levels of serotonin have been associated with impulsive behaviour and depression. Eating sugary foods and simple carbohydrates (bread, pasta, etc.) that quickly break down in the body can give a feeling of comfort, which temporarily makes you feel better.

Sensitivity

Certain individuals (including many ADHD sufferers) appear to be 'carbohydrate sensitive'. This means that their blood-sugar levels rise faster after eating than they should, causing excessive insulin to be produced in response (for more on insulin and glucose, see Chapter 10). This release of insulin in turn causes the blood-sugar levels to drop rapidly, which can leave you craving another sugary treat.

Now if we put these three words together we have a recipe for disaster. Carbohydrate sensitivity, which itself may be caused by the slow processing of glucose in the brains of ADHD sufferers, together with low levels of endorphin and serotonin, can put the sugar junkie on a roller-coaster ride of sugar highs and lows which of course will be mirrored by excessive mood swings. Unfortunately, we live in a sugar culture where there seems to be an unconscious need to add sugar to everything. Apart from providing energy (calories), sugar has no nutritional value whatsoever and yet manufacturers and many people feel the need to add spoonfuls whenever they can. Whereas essential fatty acids are by definition essential (you cannot survive without them), natural sugars, such as those in fruit and milk, are found in abundance in a well-balanced diet and do not need to be supplemented.

Time and again, when I suggest changes to the diet of children visiting the clinic, the mothers will say at the time or call me later saying, 'As he can't have sugar can he have honey instead?' or, 'If I make my own biscuits or cakes is that OK?' It has been suggested that because breast milk is sweet we develop a sweet tooth to ensure that we eat energy-producing foods. Be that as it may, what we do not need in our diets are foods that are processed too quickly, producing blood-sugar highs and lows. What we need to do is establish a sensible pattern of what we eat and when we eat it so that the needs of our bodies are met at the right time. Bad eating habits that start in childhood will continue to have a negative impact in adulthood. But it's never too late to ring the changes and by following the dietary guidelines given later in the book you too can bring about positive health changes and feel better about yourself.

Are artificial sweeteners the answer?

There are times in life when most of us think that we need to shed a pound or two, and artificial sweeteners would appear to be very helpful as part of a calorie-controlled diet. Just think about it, all the sweetness you could possibly want and virtually no added calories. Now let's stop and think for a moment: are there any possible unwanted side effects to such a choice?

Of all the artificial sweeteners, aspartame and saccharine have received the most attention and have generated a great deal of negative press. To date, approaching one hundred potential adverse reactions or side effects to aspartame consumption have been listed.

The solution to the sugar problem

Although sugar addiction itself is brain based, you can make a positive decision to change what you eat, and with a little self-discipline you will feel the difference in no time. It is important to realise that it is not just *what* you eat that is important but also *when* you eat. Breakfast is my favourite meal of the day – it's literally a golden opportunity to 'break the fast' and therefore should be the most important meal. Having not eaten for twelve hours or more the fuel tanks are empty and we need to take on board a healthy mix of proteins, fats and carbohydrates. Unfortunately, a huge advertising campaign, directed principally at children and ladies who feel they need to diet, tells us constantly that what we should be eating for breakfast is processed carbohydrates. The problem with this is that in a very short space of time the body has dealt with this processed food and is ready for the next carbohydrate fix. We will discuss what you should eat and why a little later.

TRY THE SWEET-TOOTH CHECK LIST

Answer Yes or No to the following questions:

- Do you eat sweets/chocolate most days?
- Are you fond of cereals/bread/pasta?
- Do you drink a little more than you should?
- Have you ever used recreational drugs?
- Are you overweight?
- Are you ever depressed/worried?
- Do you get stressed?
- Do you 'lose it' at times?
- Is there a family history of any of the above?

How did you do? The more 'Yes' answers, the more likely that there could be a problem.

Additives and supplements

The Mental Health Foundation report *Feeding the Mind* stated that we consume in the region of 8 to 9 pounds (4kg) of additives a year and few if any adults obtain enough of the omega-3 essential fatty acids through their diet. The report cited this as a possible causative factor in many conditions including ADHD in adults. What I believe they were suggesting and what I firmly believe is that a diet supplemented with up to 9lb of assorted chemicals and insufficient omega-3 to keep the brain healthy prevents the brain from functioning as it should and perpetuates a problem that started way back in childhood.

It is not too late to ring the changes; from the results obtained to date with adults I have treated I know this to be true. By following the dietary advice in this book, taking the appropriate food supplements every day and carrying out some simple exercises in the privacy of your own home you can make a real difference to how you think and feel. Also, you can take the eye tests and if necessary the home therapy to get them working as they should.

Case History: Mrs Smith

Mrs Smith was not a happy lady. She had brought her two sons to the clinic to be assessed and by the time they left I too had all but lost the will to live. Both the boys had a typical history of birth trauma/foetal distress, delays in attaining their developmental milestones, hyperactivity and underachievement at school. On examination both showed signs of underfunctioning of the brain's left cerebellum and the right cortex. When their eye movements were assessed using a computer-generated test, they both demonstrated convergence failure.

I sent them away with a diet sheet, a list of supplements to be taken daily and a couple of balancing exercises to be perfected. When I saw them some six weeks later their diet was still a nutritionist's nightmare, the supplements had not been taken and clearly the exercises had not even been attempted let alone perfected. Clearly the frustration and disappointment I felt must have shown on my face. Mrs Smith, now close to tears, instead of spouting the torrent of excuses I was expecting, simply said she could not cope. Her husband had gone off two years ago, since when things had gone from bad to worse. Fortunately for me, at this point Mrs Smith started talking about her childhood and asked me if I would consider seeing her for an assessment.

Mrs Smith's case history and examination results were almost identical to those of her sons. She had been born by emergency Caesarean section due to foetal distress, was late attaining most of her developmental milestones and at school had struggled to learn to read, hated spelling tests and had the attention span of a gnat. She had been in constant trouble at school and at home due to her inability to organise anything or remain focused for more than a millisecond.

What I needed here was commitment. If I was going to be able to do anything at all to help Mrs Smith, let alone the boys, she was going to have to follow the treatment regime to the letter. The starting point had to be the diet and supplements. Currently, they were all eating a diet based on processed foods laced with fizzy drinks. While carbohydrates ruled, fruit and veg figured nowhere in this recipe for disaster and Mrs Smith alone could down close to two litres of a well-known fizzy drink a day.

Away she went again, this time promising to stick to the diet, buy fresh fruit and veg and start cooking from scratch. I cannot say I was in the least bit confident of the outcome but I tried to be. When I saw them again two months later, the boys were calm and actually managed to sit still during the entire consultation, while Mrs Smith had a smile a mile wide. The diet was in place, the supplements were being taken and the exercises had become a matter of personal pride. Obviously the boys were better but the change in their mother was quite remarkable. She said that it was like the haze had cleared and she could now see; not only was she calmer but for the first time in her life she felt in control.

Over a period of several months the Smiths took on new exercises, computer-generated treatment for their eyes' convergence failure and other programmes designed to stimulate the right side of their brains. The boys remained calm and, I have to say, a pleasure to be with, and also started to achieve at school. Mrs Smith apparently met Mr Right and when last seen in the clinic was a different woman.

COULD IT BE YOU?

Take a look at the list below to see if you recognise any of these traits, and answer Yes or No to the questions. Don't worry if there are rather a lot of 'Yes' boxes ticked off. The first step towards gaining help is to realise there is a problem. Later on we can look at lots of different things that can be done to help.

- Do you have problems with paperwork?
- Do you have problems finishing work?
- Do you have poor focus/does your mind wander?
- Are you easily distracted?
- Do you have poor time management?
- Are you often late for work/appointments?
- Are you forever losing things?
- Are you forgetful?

- Do you talk nonstop?
- Are you often irritable?
- Are you impulsive/rash?
- Do you change jobs frequently?
- Are you often in debt/poor with money?
- Do you drive too fast and have had accidents?
- Do you feel calm inside?

Perfect answer = 1 yes only, to the last question

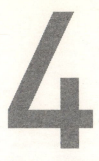

OBSESSIVE-COMPULSIVE DISORDER

WHAT IS OBSESSIVE-COMPULSIVE DISORDER?

OCD Action says:

> Obsessive Compulsive Disorder (OCD) is the name given to a condition in which people experience repetitive and upsetting thoughts and/or behaviours.

> OCD has two main features: obsessions and compulsions.

Obsessions are involuntary thoughts, images or impulses. Common obsessions include (but are not limited to) fears about dirt, germs and contamination; fears of acting out violent or aggressive thoughts or impulses; unreasonable fears of harming others, especially loved ones; abhorrent, blasphemous or sexual thoughts; inordinate concern with order, arrangement or symmetry; inability to discard useless or worn-out possessions; and fears that things are not safe, e.g. household appliances. The main features of obsessions are that they are automatic, frequent, upsetting or distressing, and difficult to control.

Just as with obsessions, there are many types of compulsions. It is common for people to carry out a compulsion in order to reduce the anxiety they feel from an obsession. Common compulsions include excessive washing and cleaning; checking; repetitive actions such as touching, counting, arranging and ordering; hoarding;

ritualistic behaviours that lessen the chances of provoking an obses-sion (e.g. putting all sharp objects out of sight); and acts which reduce obsessional fears.

Old Misunderstandings

OCD had its origins in the realms of spirituality and morality rather than medicine and it is perhaps for this reason that it is so poorly understood today.

Worries, doubts and superstitions are part of most people's lives, and obsessions and minor tics are so common in childhood they are considered a normal stage of development. When we hit a bad patch in life – such as major financial worries or divorce – we are all prone to repetitive thoughts that go round and round in our heads. The inability in these situations to get the thoughts out of your head is called perseveration. Fortunately, this usually only happens when we hit a really grim episode of our life, but imagine what it would be like if these thoughts were with you every day and night.

Some rituals – bedtime routines or religious practices – are a comfort and form an important part of a great many people's lives. Some obsessive traits are carried over from childhood into adulthood and are built into a person's personality. One day I was talking to a mother about her daughter's problems and mentioned aspects of obsessive behaviour. The mother was uncertain as to what I was talk-ing about and asked what I meant. To give an example I described a fairly typical example of a woman who organises her larder with mil-itary precision. Every tin has to be arranged by size and content, with the label facing forward, and God help anyone who disrupts the order. At this point her daughter interrupted and said, 'That's you, Mummy.' This brings us to another commonly asked question, namely, 'Is it genetic?'

A Genetic Obsession?

To date no specific gene or genes for obsessive-compulsive disorder have been identified and I don't believe there ever will be. As we will see a little later, OCD is associated with tics, disorders and other learn-ing/behavioural problems, which makes it far more likely (along with the other learning/behavioural difficulties) that the problem is with the timing of brain development.

Certainly childhood-onset OCD does run in families and, as with all the learning/behavioural problems, a child is more likely to go on to develop problems if there is a family history. In this situation there is a raised probability of developing a feature of OCD behaviour, not 'inheriting' a specific activity. By that I mean that a mother with a compulsion to wash her hands incessantly may have a child who becomes obsessed with a ritual that does not involve washing.

It has been suggested that the neurotransmitter serotonin might be the underlying cause. This is backed up by the way that serotonin re-uptake inhibitors (drugs which prevent serotonin from being removed from where it acts) work so well in treating OCD. The neurotransmitter dopamine could also be involved.

Just How Common Is OCD?

In the USA it has been estimated that one in fifty adults have OCD. However, twice that many may have bouts of OCD behavioural traits at times in their lives when they are under increased stress. In the UK the figure has been put at 1 to 2 per cent of the population.

NORMAL SIGNS – EVERYBODY CAN HAVE THESE

In childhood
- Bedtime rituals
- Sticking to preferred routines
- Obsessions with collecting and/or certain subjects e.g. dinosaurs
- Items in their room must be in the exact same place

In adults
- Recurrent thoughts
- Having to read and re-read signs/adverts, etc.
- Having to double-check that you locked the door, etc.
- Fearing that you might do something very bad

ABNORMAL SIGNS – SEEN IN OCD

Obsessions
- Perseveration – cyclic thoughts

- Abnormal fear of germs/dirt
- Fear of losing control – harming self or others
- Aggressive or sexual urges

Compulsion
- Repeated physical or mental acts – e.g. handwashing, number sequences
- Following strict rules
- Rituals – that are very time-consuming
- Having to check and double-check, again and again

Anxiety and emotions

It is of interest to note that a certain Dr Benedict-Augustin Morel (1809–73) considered OCD a disease of the emotions, which he believed originated from the autonomic nervous system (the part of the nervous system that controls 'automatic' things like the heart rate, blood pressure, digestion, etc.). His belief was based on his observations that the obsessions and compulsions were accompanied by anxiety. This was a very astute observation as it came long before the work of the French physician Paul Broca in 1878 and James Papez in 1937, both of whom described models of emotion.

The degree of anxiety and symptoms such as increased heart rate, blood pressure and sweating, associated with developmental delay (which includes OCD and Tourette's syndrome) is still often not considered, so sadly many people fail to appreciate the true suffering of someone with OCD.

Rest and Digest vs Fight or Flight

Tucked away in the base of the brain just in front of the brainstem is a tiny area (weighing just 4 grams) called the hypothalamus. Although small, it has the all-important role of controlling such vital functions as core body temperature, hunger, thirst, oxygen levels in the blood and the desire to mate. It is connected to the body's organs via a chain of nerve cells which make up the autonomic nervous system.

The autonomic nervous system can be divided into three parts.

The **parasympathetic division** aids digestion, slows the heart rate and helps you breathe easily. Hence it is said to have a 'rest and digest' function.

The **enteric division** controls the digestive system. It can work independently but its functions are altered by the other two divisions.

The **sympathetic division** stops digestion, speeds up breathing and the heart rate, pushes up blood pressure and in extreme conditions empties the bladder and bowels. It should function only in states of great danger and hence has been said to have a 'fight or flight' function. It is, needless to say, associated with a great deal of sweating.

You can see that if the sympathetic nervous system starts working when it shouldn't, then a whole host of unpleasant things are going to happen to you. Apart from having a digestive system that is constantly in effect being turned on and off, the stress hormone cortisol will be released, which can play havoc with your immune (body's defence mechanism) system and you are going to be in constant panic mode.

So what could cause this to happen? To explain this we will have to look at how various parts of the brain work and how these various regions interact.

More Brain Mapping

We have already mentioned (in Chapter 3) the anterior cingulate that lies on the dark side of the brain and the infraorbital area above the eyes. Between these two areas is another small area called the perigenual area. The perigenual area has many jobs to do but importantly here it appears to have a very important role in controlling the sympathetic nervous system – switching it on, and also integrating emotions into our movements.

This first function helps to explain why so many people with aspects of developmental delay are anxious, constantly on edge and often have cold, wet hands and smelly feet.

This is because the two areas on either side of the perigenual area feed into it and therefore have a great impact upon its level of function. One of these areas that feeds in is the infraorbital area, which deals with the social graces (how to behave), and also has a role in how we feel – happy or sad. The anterior cingulate area helps control our level of activity and our ability to focus.

The dark side of the brain – internal wall

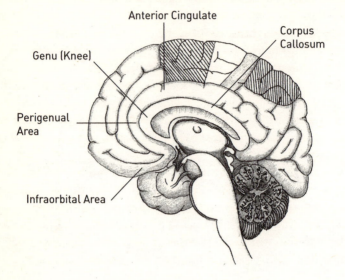

The second function, put simply, is to add whatever emotion you are feeling to the movement you are going to perform, and determine *how* you are going to do it. If someone passes a newborn baby to you, you are going to have to be very careful and gentle so as not to harm the infant. On the other hand, if you are in a situation where your life is at risk you are going to have to be as strong and violent as you can be.

In order to get a better understanding as to how OCD and tics can occur, we need to describe some of the 'loops' that exist in the brain that allow us to move.

Circles in the Mind

Buried deep within the brain on each side is a tightly packed collection of brain cells known together as the basal nuclei and the thalamus.

There are five basic loops that involve these structures providing for things like eye movements and desired controlled movements. If we look at just one such loop we can see not only what is meant to happen but also what can happen when things go wrong.

A circle in the mind

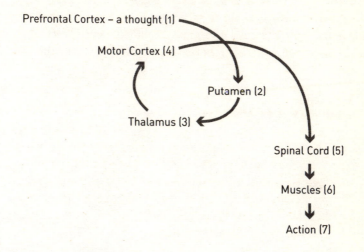

A moving experience

Let us suppose that something very sad has happened – your football team just lost 4–0 – and you are moved to tears. You need to reach for your hankie and wipe the tears from your eyes. To do this you have to send a positive message from a region of the brain called the frontal cortex down to another, using a neurotransmitter. The second region then sends a negative message to yet another brain region, blocking it from doing what it was before. Since it was previously stopping the region of the brain that causes movement from working, this negative message effectively tells the 'motor cortex' (the brain's movement centre) to work, and it in turn sends messages down the spinal cord to make the necessary muscles move – and wipe away those tears.

Escape

Let us now consider what happens if the brain, particularly on the right side, does not mature and develop as it should and the frontal cortex produces messages when it shouldn't. Basically, depending on which of the five primary loops are involved, you will get involuntary movements (tics) or thoughts that you cannot get out of your mind (obsessions). As most of these problems start fairly early on in childhood while the brain is still growing, or when we are suffering high levels of stress, this seems to be a very plausible explanation.

Also, because there are far more von Economo cells on the right side of the brain there is a greater probability of developmental delay being associated with the right side – and this is generally the case.

Letter from an OCD sufferer

As a child OCD was very evident in my life – washing my hands repeatedly right up to the elbow and later whilst playing football for the school team I developed a ritual of tapping the left foot three times and then the right foot three times. This became so intense that the last thing I wanted was to receive the ball. Later still the rituals became more introverted, such as mental rituals that had to be repeated over and over to avoid harm coming to my loved ones or others – up to three hundred times a day or more.

Throughout my school days I had intense difficulty grasping the formula of a subject that my fellow students found easy. Once a subject was grasped I would leave the others standing. However, because of the feeling of inadequacy and peer pressure I covered the fact that I couldn't grasp subjects and fell further and further behind. To compensate for this I was the class comedian (though inside I was really hurting). Consequently this brought trouble my way and I was constantly in detention every week.

Throughout my whole life I suffered terrible depression and anxiety that necessitated regular medication, which left me terribly tired and unable to function. Also I suffered from Seasonal Affective Disorder (SAD) and the winter was a dreadful time with our climate. My moaning about the weather drove my wife to distraction. However, one day I happened to come across a middle-page spread in a national newspaper about your work which touched a chord in me and after reading your book *Is That My Child?* it was a revelation that someone knew me intimately on the inside (something that sadly psychiatrists and psychologists failed to understand and this led to my breakdown). Also, whilst reading your book I saw a list of nine behavioural descriptive symptoms of ADD with a rider that if your child has six or more it would be considered to be suffering from ADD – I had all nine! Hence the inability to grasp subjects.

In view of the foregoing, I embarked on the Tinsley House treatment and twelve months later (although for me at the age of 61 it will take longer than a child) I can truly say I have never felt better in all my life – no depression (off all antidepressants) the intensity of OCD has dropped dramatically by 85 per cent and absolutely no SAD, in fact my wife moans when there is prolonged rain and I say 'Never mind, don't let it get you down, dear' – what a role reversal!

I only wish this treatment had been available fifty years before but this has given my later years of life a quality I never believed possible, for which I am eternally grateful to you.

P.S. You could add that your treatment has lifted a veil from my mind to allow far better grasping of new subjects that OCD prevented.

Anthony Whaley

TOURETTE'S SYNDROME – TIC DISORDERS

What is a tic?

A tic is an involuntary movement. A muscle or group of muscles move – tic – when you don't want them to or you make a noise or grunt rather like the throat-clearing some people do when they get nervous.

Tics can be divided into four categories. You can have:

1) **A transient tic,** which can be a movement or making a noise that lasts for more than four weeks but less than twelve.
2) **A chronic tic,** which is either a movement or a sound (but not both) that is present for more than a year.
3) **Tourette's syndrome,** which is movement and sounds together for more than a year.
4) **A tic disorder (not otherwise specified)** that does not fit into any of the other categories.

A TOURETTE'S GENE?

As OCD traits and minor tics are so common in childhood they are considered a normal stage of development, it's surprising that scientists are still looking for a Tourette's gene as opposed to thinking that tics could be a sign that the normal development of the brain is having a little hiccough. When you consider that as many as one child in five goes through a phase of having a tic disorder, and they usually pass through it without any signs remaining, it does make you think that maybe the geneticists are barking up the wrong tree.

The caricature of Tourette's

The classic picture of Tourette's syndrome often seen portrayed in films is the exception rather than the rule. The vast majority of children and adults (often the parents) have a variety of minor motor (movement) tics and/or vocal tics. In the past year I have only seen one patient that let fly an expletive.

Control at a price

Although these motor and vocal tics are described as involuntary movements (you can't control them), they can to a certain extent be held back. Some sufferers can stop the tics for a period of time and release them when they are in the privacy of their own home. Therefore, it can come as something of a surprise for a teacher or employer to learn that a child or employee has a tic disorder. Some sufferers can disguise their tics by building them into what might be considered to be normal movements. However, holding back tics or indeed OCD rituals comes at a cost. Often when the child gets home his or her behaviour can become very disturbed or they suffer terrible guilt when they finally have to give in to the overwhelming urge.

A BIT OF HISTORY – GILLES DE LA TOURETTE

Tourette's syndrome was originally described by Gilles de la Tourette as *'maladie des tics convulsifs avec coprolalie'* (an illness of convulsive tics with the involuntary use of obscene words). The early documented cases of Tourette's syndrome were of adult patients and it was not until the 1930s that the tics were described in normal children. However, Tourette did note that as well as the involuntary movement tics, vocal tics and swearing, the disorder began in childhood, (usually between seven and ten years of age), affected males more than females and was, in his opinion, hereditary. He also noted that the tics usually started in the face or upper extremities and that the symptoms waxed and waned and were made worse by stress.

Common Signs of Tourette's

- Excessive blinking
- Head-turning
- Throat-clearing
- Grimacing
- Grunting
- Squeaking
- One-sided facial tics
- Eyes rolling up

The cause of Tourette's

The exact cause of Tourette's syndrome is unknown, but it appears to be linked to the gene or genes that control certain neurotransmitters, notably dopamine and serotonin. I believe the reason why Tourette's syndrome is so poorly understood is because, like OCD, ADHD etc., it is still thought to be a condition in its own right. Once we look at the pattern in which these so-called conditions appear, it becomes clear that we are dealing with a group of symptoms that together form a developmental delay – and not with individual conditions.

Where these symptoms begin not only goes a long way towards explaining the underlying cause but also presents an opportunity to provide effective treatment.

About a third of people with the disorder have relatives with Tourette's syndrome, while another third have family members with milder tic disorders. There is also more obsessive-compulsive disorder and attention deficit hyperactivity disorder in families of people with Tourette's syndrome.

Also, because Tourette's is much more frequent in men, the role of hormones has been considered and it has been suggested that the male foetus might be vulnerable to a spike in the female hormone oestrogen from the mother, during a specific stage of pregnancy.

Symptoms in patterns

I believe that none of the learning and behavioural disabilities should be viewed in isolation and, rather than pigeonhole people into the box that appears to fit best, it would be far more sensible to consider these conditions as *symptoms* that occur in various patterns.

I prefer the term developmental delay as it allows each person's unique symptoms to be considered. The unique symptom patterns also provide a clue as to factors beyond genetics that play a role in causing developmental delay.

When researching Tourette's syndrome, time and again it is associated with OCD, along with ADHD. However, in a recent study the association between these three conditions (symptoms) was also strongly linked to the other so-called learning/behavioural problems. Hence my insistence that these supposed conditions are no more than symptoms. Furthermore, when looking at the research into the underlying cause of so many of these 'conditions', the same neurotransmitters keep cropping up, as do specific areas of the brain.

- Dyspraxia is strongly associated with learning disabilities, emotional problems, oppositional defiance and ADHD.
- Dyslexia is strongly associated with Tourette's syndrome and OCD.
- ADHD is found to be associated with dyslexia, OCD, Tourette's syndrome and dyspraxia.

PRACTICAL ADVICE

What makes tics and ritual worse?

- Just talking about a person's tics – or habits as they are often called – in front of them can set off motor (movement) tics in seconds.

- Being overtired can make a big difference to the occurrence of tics. Children are often worse at the end of term.
- Lack of sleep can cause an upsurge in symptoms.
- Drinking alcohol can make symptoms worse the next day.
- Stress is certainly a big factor. In children the build-up to exams or in adults the period leading up to a big presentation can see an increase in symptoms.
- Diet has been implicated on numerous occasions. The Mental Health Foundation has suggested that food additives and insufficient omega-3 can play a role in the generation of anxiety and signs of ADHD.

What helps reduce tics and ritual?

- Being distracted by something enjoyable or engaging in an activity (such as playing the piano) can see a complete cessation of tics.
- Getting enough sleep and taking exercise in the fresh air can help prevent a build-up.
- Taking alcohol in moderation – just a little of what you fancy does you good.
- A healthy diet as free from artificial sweeteners and additives as possible has been shown to help.
- Supplementing your diet with omega-3 (see Chapter 11) can provide significant benefits.

Developmental Delay and IQ

I have often been asked if developmental delay is associated with a low IQ. Often people assume that if you can't read and have handwriting that looks like it has been produced by a spider, then clearly you are not too bright.

The ability to learn depends on a couple of things: one is the brain you are born with and the second is the ability to learn. One thing that we know for certain is that we are not all born equal. During the process of growth and development something called apoptosis – programmed cell death – takes place in the brain. What happens is that literally millions of brain cells develop from an area of the developing brain called neuroepithelium. As these cells develop, they have to move off to where they are destined to live; once they arrive they make contact with other brain cells. In order to survive they must migrate to the right location and make contact with other cells. Those cells that get lost en route or fail to make contact die and the number of cells that don't make it can vary considerably. You might lose 10, 20, 30, or 50 per cent. Obviously, the number of cells you lose will impact upon the processing ability of your brain. Anyone who knows about computers will tell you that a modern computer will far outstrip a computer from just ten years ago in terms of not only processing speed but also how much it can do at once and the size of its memory. To a certain extent the brain functions in a similar way: fewer cells equal reduced processing capabilities.

Let us suppose that you went through the process of apoptosis and came out of it with a good few brains cells intact. So far so good, but the development of the brain is not over yet. Although a great many people assume that the brain is complete at birth and just needs to get bigger, they are wrong. Four months after birth the second generation of brain cells – von Economo cells, gigantopyramidal cells, etc. – come into their own right. You may have done very well for yourself during apoptosis but without a successful passage through bpoptosis – when the second-generation cells develop, move and make contact with other cells – you will be less able to use the intelligence you have been gifted to its best advantage.

Therefore, you could have the potential brainpower to do really well in life but without the ability to use that function it is a struggle to learn, to get the education you deserve and be able to fulfil your potential. As we will see later, without the necessary education you can fail in so many aspects of life, not just in terms of income and the knock-on effects that can have, but also in terms of personal relationships.

It's not all doom and gloom – disadvantages can be overcome!

Thousands of people struggle to read or think they are dyslexic, when in fact they have secondary dyslexia – an inability to control their eyes for close vision – which in most people can be fixed in a matter of weeks. Helping the brain to grow and develop in children is so very easy and so it is with adults if they simply follow a plan designed to help the brain function as it should.

I can't promise that you will become a genius overnight but you can take very positive steps to achieve the best that you can be and attain your potential.

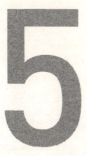

AUTISM AND ASPERGER'S SYNDROME

WHAT IS AUTISM?

The National Autistic Society (UK) says:

Autism is a lifelong developmental disability that affects the way a person communicates and relates to people around them. Children and adults with autism have difficulties with everyday social interaction. Their ability to develop friendships is generally limited as is their capacity to understand other people's emotional expression.

People with autism can often have accompanying learning disabilities but everyone with the condition shares a difficulty in making sense of the world.

The Autism Society of America says:

Autism is a complex developmental disability that typically appears during the first three years of life and is the result of a neurological disorder that affects the normal functioning of the brain, impacting development in the areas of social interaction and communication skills. Both children and adults with autism typically show difficulties in verbal and non-verbal communication, social interactions, and leisure or play activities. One should keep in mind however, that autism is a spectrum disorder and it affects each individual differently and at varying degrees – this is why early diagnosis is so crucial. By learning the signs, a child can begin benefiting from one of the many specialised intervention programmes.

THE HISTORY OF AUTISM AND ASPERGER'S SYNDROME

The word autism was coined by the psychiatrist Eugen Bleuler in 1911, and comes from the Greek word *autos*, meaning 'self', which is perhaps the very embodiment of the condition. However, it was not until 1938 that Leo Kanner applied the term to describe the behaviour of eleven children in his care at the Johns Hopkins Hospital. These children had until this time been considered as being intellectually impaired and/or emotionally disturbed.

Six years later Hans Asperger described children in his care that, although appearing to be of normal intelligence, lacked social skills, didn't demonstrate levels of empathy appropriate for their age and were clumsy.

AUTISTIC SPECTRUM DISORDER

NHS Direct's Health encyclopaedia says:

Autistic spectrum disorder is the term that is used to describe a group of disorders, including autism and Asperger's syndrome. The word 'spectrum' is used because the characteristics of the condition vary from one person to another. Those with autism may also have a learning disability. Those who have Asperger's syndrome tend to have average, or above average, intelligence, but still have difficulty making sense of the world.

So it would appear that autism is the result of a developmental problem of the brain that starts early on in life and affects people differently but has a major impact on social interactions – fitting into society.

Autism is one of five separate disorders that fall within a group of conditions called pervasive developmental disorders. Sufferers have real problems with making sense of the world around them and therefore fitting into it. However, these definitions do not tell us what really causes autism, what it is or what can be done to help. In fact in many ways they are so vague as to make you think that yet again square pegs are being fitted into round holes.

The five disorders under pervasive developmental disorders are:

- Autistic Disorder
- Asperger's Disorder
- Autistic Spectrum Disorders
- Childhood Disintegrative Disorder (CDD)
- Rett's Disorder (now generally not included)

Traits of autism

The characteristics or traits of autism can vary from person to person and this is why it's described as a 'spectrum disorder'. It is my belief that we should apply the label autistic only if someone has *all* the diagnostic criteria. If they don't, we should say that the person has autistic traits as part of a developmental delay syndrome. I will explain my reasoning later but for now we must consider just what the characteristics of autism are. They can be divided into three main areas:

- social interaction
- communication
- imagination

Mix and match

A person who has what is described as 'autism' may find it hard to relate to other people.

Parents find that their child:

- Resists physical contact/shuns affection
- Makes poor eye contact or avoids eye contact
- Is detached in their own little world
- Prefers to be alone
- Plays on the periphery if at all

Others find that the child:

- Has little or no interest in other people
- Are difficult to befriend

- Lack basic social skills
- Cannot read other people's emotions and often can't control their own

Talking and listening

A person with 'autism' may have problems not only with verbal communication – using words and sentences to convey what they want or need – but also may be unable to pick up on the nonverbal clues that we all use to get our message across.

Talking and listening:

- **Talking** – we need to use the right words in the right order to show what we mean.
- **Listening** – we need to understand what has been said plus pick up on the tone of voice and inflections used.

Visual communication:

- **Reading** facial expressions – 'I can see that you are upset'.
- **Understanding** gestures and postures – 'You seem tense'.

Imaginative play

Children in particular with 'autism' often lack imaginative play and cannot create a play situation using objects around them. They will often play the same game over and over again or watch the same video or part of a video constantly. This lack of imaginative play and the inability to form friendships limits the child's ability to develop.

The overloaded brain

Day and night, but particularly by day, the brain receives a constant flood of information from the senses. The eyes, ears, nose and skin, plus our joints and muscles and internal organs send millions of tiny messages up the spinal cord, into the brainstem or directly into the brain itself. There are so many messages in fact that the brain would not be able to cope with such a massive amount of input, and there are filters to reduce and prioritise this deluge of sensory information. It is mainly the spinal cord and the region of the brain called the thalamus that filter out trivial input so that only important information reaches the brain's cortex for processing.

View of the left side of the brain

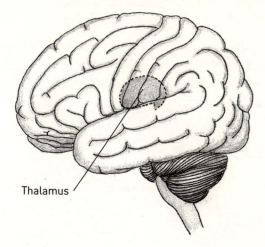

Thalamus

Imagine how it would be if you were constantly aware that every item of clothing you are wearing is touching your skin. At times we are all aware of an itchy label or, particularly when we are tired, can be annoyed by just our shirt touching our back. If you have ever had the misfortune to stay in a hotel just before Christmas you will have experienced the torture of half-heard music from some firm's pre-Christmas office party that prevents you from sleeping for hours.

Many people with 'autism' (and other developmental delays to a certain extent) can be oversensitive to things such as touch, textures, bright lights and sound. This means that a child taken to nursery school for the first time may disappear under a table or cover their ears to block out the noise. Many children will only wear certain clothes and become very difficult to feed, as they will only eat foods with the 'right' taste and texture.

How common is 'autism'?

Not so long ago the estimated figures for autism would have been around one or two cases per thousand births. Now if you surf the net you will find statements such as:

- 'Autism is the most common of the Pervasive Developmental Disorders, affecting an estimated 1 in 150 births in the USA.'

- 'Recent research in the UK suggests that around 1 in 100 people have Autistic Spectrum Disorder and it is said to affect four times as many males than females.'

Some researchers have suggested that the increase in the number of children diagnosed as having 'autism' is thanks to better diagnosis, but even if this were true, it doesn't explain the dramatic increase that has taken place since the 1980s, and some observers are now saying that 'autism' has now reached epidemic proportions.

What causes 'autism'?

The cause of 'autism' is unknown. However, research (yet again) suggests that genetics may be involved, and there is also some evidence to show that the condition may be linked to environmental factors, such as pollution, poisoning or infection during pregnancy.

To date an 'autism' gene has yet to be identified and again I must say that I doubt if one ever will be found, as I believe the problem is that the timing of the development of the brain is at fault. One interesting line of thought is that the chemical signposts within the developing brain may fail to develop as they should, and so migrating brain cells get lost en route to their destination. It has been suggested that things such as severe viral infections in the pregnant mother may mean that the 'signposts' in her developing baby's brain fail to be established.

Finding a theory of autism

Professor John Allman and Esther Nimchinsky rediscovered the early work of von Economo and went on to study both the structure and migration patterns of these late-developing cells. Recently Allman has suggested that von Economo cells are *absent* in autism, and that this might be the underlying cause of the condition. Since that time further research has questioned his results. More studies using a much bigger sample size will be required to provide a definitive answer.

However, I believe that it is these second-generation cells that help make us what we are, allowing our innate intelligence to shine forth and provide us with all that we consider to be human. If John Allman's suggestion proves to be correct, then a total absence of von Economo cells would be the cause of true autism, while a developmental delay in the maturation of the cells would produce autistic traits. A theory like this would explain why people's autistic traits across the spectrum are so individual, and would also do away with the ever-increasing and changing diagnostic pigeonholes we are meant to force people into.

Bpoptosis and 'autism'

Bpoptosis is the term I first used in 2005 to describe how the second-generation brain cells develop, migrate and make contact with other cells. Of the second generation of brain cells we know that the von Economo cells should end up – migrate to – the anterior cingulate on the dark side of the brain and the infraorbital area just above the eyes. Until fairly recently not a lot was known about these two areas. Although our knowledge is far from complete we now know a lot more about them, and it all fits in perfectly with both the possible cause and consequence of developmental delay.

The anterior cingulate region:

- Is involved in tasks involving complex thinking (see ADD)
- Is more active in anxiety, phobic states and OCD
- Is less active in ADHD

The infraorbital prefrontal cortex is involved in:

- Self-control appropriate to a person's age
- The social graces – fitting into society

If Allman's suggestion is true and my theories prove to be correct, then a pattern of developmental delay based on the severity of symptoms would go a long way to explain why the appearance and symptoms of the various so-called learning/behavioural problems are so varied and individual. It would also explain why they will always appear in comorbidity (together).

1) No von Economo cells = True autism
2) Severely delayed von Economo cells = Some autistic traits
3) Moderately delayed von Economo cells = Severe learning/behavioural problems
4) Slightly delayed von Economo cells = Minor to moderate learning/behavioural problems

Looking in the right place

If we now consider all the 'conditions' we have looked at so far as being no more than symptoms and place these symptoms in the categories above, we can see a clear picture of what is happening.

We no longer need to pigeonhole people into ill-fitting categories – we can now look at the complete and unique symptoms that each individual sufferer must have and by doing this understand how much developmental delay they have. If we can diagnose the problem accurately, and know where it comes from, the potential to fix it suddenly becomes available to us.

With pretty well all the conditions we have talked about so far, scientists have searched for a specific gene or genes for each 'condition'. But now we can say that they are symptoms, not conditions, and symptoms that will always appear together, as part of a developmental delay syndrome. This means that instead of looking for the autism gene, scientists can concentrate on the genes that specifically control the late development of the brain – bpoptosis.

Time and again (and no more is this true than of 'autism'), environmental factors, pollution, food additives, maternal stress and foetal distress have been suggested as possible factors in causing these 'conditions'. Now, armed with the knowledge of the way genes can be switched on or off, we can begin to see that anything that stresses the individual during critical windows of development could perhaps leave some or all bpoptosis genes switched off. This knowledge alone gives us the potential to consider ways that we can flick the switches and thereby kick-start the development and maturation of the second-generation cells, which I believe are vital to the optimum functioning of the brain.

ASPERGER'S SYNDROME

People with Asperger's are often described as 'high-functioning' autistic. They generally do not have a learning disability and are often of average or above-average intelligence. They will usually have fewer problems with spoken language but experience difficulties with social communication – this is because they have a total inability to interpret or even notice the facial and body-language signs given off by others.

TEENAGERS AND TESTOSTERONE

It is interesting to note that this inability to read nonverbal communication is a normal developmental stage, particularly in teenage boys when the levels of the male hormone testosterone start to rise. Generally this is short-lived and is thought to be due to the brain's prefrontal cortex, which is normally used to read facial expressions, being otherwise occupied trying to control the region of the brain called the hypothalamus. The hypothalamus functions in controlling many of our bodily functions including the desire to mate. When testosterone kicks in, boys start being very interested in girls, and as a boy's prefrontal cortex can't be expected to do too many things at the same time, it loses its ability to see that his mother is about to blow a gasket because he is late for the school run and yet again he cannot find his iPod.

Understanding how others feel

Being unable to understand what other people are feeling (in other words, a lack of empathy) is often quoted as the most dysfunctional aspect of Asperger's syndrome. The inability to sympathise with people contributes greatly to the sufferer's lack of friends and this, coupled with a complete absence of social etiquette – knowing when to speak, when to smile and when to nod approval – tends to drive people away.

Also, people with Asperger's often have a very narrow and highly specialised knowledge of a particular area of interest, and they often force this upon others in a long-winded monologue, using a monotone voice – and this makes things worse. Unlike people with autism, Asperger's sufferers are not shrinking violets and *will* approach others. However, the approach can be ill-timed, inappropriate and often resembles a bull in a china shop.

Clumsiness?

Asperger's sufferers are physically as well as mentally clumsy. Children with Asperger's are often late in attaining large and small movement skills, and the adult sufferer often has poor co-ordination, with an awkward gait and poor spatial awareness. They don't realise how close they are to other people and things, and this can lead to other people feeling uncomfortable or angry as they get too close.

Every time you move a muscle, the brain has to know what is going to happen, in order that it knows precisely where every part of your body is. Think about it – if you were sitting cross-legged but your brain had not registered the fact that you had crossed the right leg over the left and you suddenly had to get up, your brain would assume that both your feet were on the ground. Hence the expression 'falling over your own feet'.

But it doesn't end there. We tend to think of vision as 'seeing', but actually a lot of what the visual system does involves the 'non-seeing' aspects of vision. One thing the non-seeing part of the visual system has to do is detect movements at the edges of our field of vision, in case something is creeping up on us, but also to be aware of what is immediately around us. Even if you are staring at an object in front of you, you should be aware of objects that are around you and this awareness should heighten if one of these objects moves. Without this awareness you are an accident waiting to happen.

Synaesthesia – 'feeling' blue, red or purple
Many years ago, I was listening to a patient describing his symptoms. The pain in the neck, aching in the shoulder and pins-and-needles in the right arm was all making perfect sense to me. At that point he described the blue pain that accompanied the pins-and-needles in the arm and I immediately began to doubt this man's sanity. However, in my defence I had only been in practice a relatively short space of time and I did not have the benefit then of a postgraduate education in neurology. Had I but known, this man was exhibiting what is known as synaesthesia. That is, when the sensory outcome we experience gets muddled up so that we 'taste' words or 'feel' colours.

Synaesthesia is not uncommon in association with the other signs and symptoms of developmental delay.

How much is down to chance – how much can we change?
Although there may be a genetic susceptibility that runs through certain families, the evidence is accumulating that many factors within our power to control can make a huge difference. Changing the way we look at the developmental disorders can, I believe, change the fate

of thousands of people and it is within our power to help every generation to pass as smoothly as possible from childhood into adulthood without carrying the unnecessary stigma of a learning disability.

CARING AND COPING

It has been estimated that only 15 per cent of sufferers from the autistic spectrum disorders are able to leave home and function totally independently. Therefore, the vast majority of autistic adults need constant care. People with Asperger's (which is often termed high-functioning autism) may be able to hold down a job. Indeed, they may have the most amazing innovative ideas or show traits of genius, but many at the end of the day return to the care of their families and the security of the family home.

Most autistic children pass into adulthood with their condition getting little better, and generally have to live at home with their parents or in residential homes. How well an autistic adult can hold down a job, run a home, and take care of all the paperwork that comes through the post will obviously vary from individual to individual. Education and training has been shown to play a vital role, and help in the home, where available, can make it possible for others to remain independent.

It is not all doom and gloom
It has been speculated that many brilliant and famous people, working in various fields, *may* have suffered from autism or Asperger's. The list includes:

- **Authors** – Jonathan Swift, Hans Christian Andersen, Lewis Carroll, William Butler Yeats, Arthur Conan Doyle and George Orwell.
- **Philosophers** – Spinoza, Immanuel Kant and A J Ayer.
- **Musicians and composers** – Wolfgang Amadeus Mozart, Ludwig van Beethoven and Bela Bartok.
- **Artists** – Vincent van Gogh, Jack B Yeats, L S Lowry and Andy Warhol.

And would you believe that it has been suggested that even Albert Einstein himself may have had autistic traits. Clearly there is hope for us all.

Testing times

The Greater Manchester Consortium was developed to help local services deal with autism. The mini-test below is based on the GMC measure but I have added and amended it so it can be used to provide an indication as to the presence of 'autistic' traits.

PART 1 – DO YOU?

(Answer YES or NO)

1) Avoid the company of others?
2) Not share your interests?
3) Not understand other people's feeling?
4) Have problems taking turns?
5) Often interrupt people?
6) Repeat what other people say?
7) Ever rock to and fro particularly when worried?
8) Ever get obsessed with objects?

PART 2

9) Has anybody commented on the way you speak?
10) Has anybody said to you 'That's not a real word'?
11) Have you ever flapped your hands when excited?
12) Are you sensitive to noise and/or bright lights?
13) Are you a bit clumsy?
14) Are you a touch accident-prone?
15) Do you bump into things a lot?
16) Are you a bit slow dressing yourself?

PART 3 – ASK YOUR MUM

17) Did you ever walk on tiptoe?
18) Did you make poor eye contact?
19) Did you flap as a child?
20) Did you spin yourself or objects a lot?
21) Did you lack affection?
22) Were you a bit late with your milestones?
23) Did you have any little obsessions?

Now add up the total 'Yes' answers.

This mini-test is only intended to give an idea as to the presence of traits and should not be considered as being diagnostic. If your answers were mainly 'Yes' then you might want to think about having a formal assessment.

Case History: Darren

Five-year-old Darren was brought to see me by his very concerned parents. Although being born at full term his passage into the world was not an easy one and when he went into foetal distress an assisted delivery was used to hasten his arrival. He was breast-fed for only six weeks as he struggled to latch on to the nipple and was very slow to feed. It was over eight months before he could sit unaided; he did not crawl and didn't attempt to walk until he was approaching eighteen months. His speech was delayed and speech therapy was started when he was three and still barely saying half a dozen words (sounds). At five he was still wetting himself by day on a fairly regular basis and was in pull-ups at night.

His mother had attempted on several occasions to get him into local nursery schools but on each attempt Darren became so distressed that either she had taken him home or the school had suggested he should be collected. Darren had been seen by various professionals and was now considered to be on the autistic spectrum and was attending a special school. Although he had now settled into the school, he did not mix with the other children and was gaining very little by being there.

At home Darren lived a life governed by routine, any change from which would generate a mega tantrum. He played with a few toys and watched three videos and two TV programmes. His diet was very limited and mainly carbohydrate-based. He was fascinated by the swing in the garden but any attempt to place him on it or move it would result in him going rigid before screaming uncontrollably.

On direct questioning his mother stated that he flapped when excited, often walked on tiptoe and made poor eye contact. However, I noticed that as he sat cuddled up on his mother's lap he would look at me on the odd occasion and was glancing around the room. Clearly he was more than happy to be cuddled, but was he generally affectionate? The answer was a very definite yes.

Having completed the consultation it was time to attempt the examination. After completing half a dozen tests I gave up as Dar-

ren was having none of it and I was clearly wasting my time. I sent the family away with a list of dietary changes to be put in place, supplements to be provided each morning and some very simple exercises to be carried out on a daily basis. One of the exercises was to place Darren on an office chair and spin him slowly to his left three times. After the three rotations his mother was to look at his eyes to see if they were flickering from side to side. If they were not then she should spin him a further three times. This little exercise was to be performed at least three times a day.

I saw Darren again six weeks later. After a major battle the diet was more or less in place, the supplements were going down a treat and the exercises had been carried out as directed. I really did not need to ask how he was getting on as a totally different child was sitting in front of me. After two weeks on the treatment regime Darren had not only indicated that he wanted to get on the garden swing but very slowly had taken to being swung to and fro. Significantly, his speech patterns had changed and he was now making good eye contact with strangers.

Darren went from strength to strength, was soon dry day and night and, although he had a lot of catching up to do, was well on the path to being the child his parents had so much wanted. One year later he was in a mainstream school and, though still in need of a lot of extra help, was making up lost ground. We cannot say for certain what would have happened to Darren without the specific therapeutic interventions that were made. However, what we do know for certain is that the child that was once labelled as 'autistic' is now safe, happy and rapidly moving towards the best that he can be.

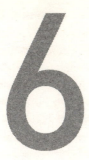

THE IMPACT OF LEARNING AND BEHAVIOURAL PROBLEMS ON THE INDIVIDUAL

Before looking at the effects that learning and behavioural disabilities can have on the individual it is necessary to look briefly at the patterns of symptoms which typically appear. Generally speaking a parent or individual will target one particular symptom or sign because it is the most obvious. You struggle to read and therefore focus on the dyslexia without really considering the fact that you are clumsy and have the attention span of a gnat. Because historically the learning/behavioural disabilities have been considered to be specific individual 'conditions' the professionals dealing with them have also focused on the main feature to the exclusion of all else. To be fair, more and more professionals are beginning to consider that these 'conditions' do appear together, but they still seem, for the most part, to be missing the point.

All these so-called 'conditions' are no more than symptoms and symptoms that will always be found in various combinations.

HOW THE SYMPTOMS COMBINE

A few years ago I carried out a simple but very useful exercise in the clinic. I took a significant number of case notes from the filing cabinets and entered into the computer such details as who had previously diagnosed the patient, what the main or primary diagnosis was, what secondary 'conditions' were apparent from the consultation/examination, whether the child was a boy or girl, and so on. I was then able to create from the figures various tables of the combinations in which the 'conditions' appeared. For example, of all the patients with a primary diagnosis of attention deficit, 20 per cent of them also had the signs and symptoms for obsessive-compulsive disorder, 18 per cent had Tourette's syndrome, 32 per cent had attention deficit hyperactivity disorder and 86 per cent had dyspraxia.

The full results were as follows:

Primary diagnosis dyslexia
84% also had dyspraxia
62% also had ADD
21% also had ADHD
16% also had OCD
6% also had Tourette's

Primary diagnosis dyspraxia
70% also had ADD
50% also had dyslexia
36% also had ADHD
21% also had OCD
17% also had Tourette's

Primary diagnosis ADHD
89% also had dyspraxia
64% also had ADD
30% also had dyslexia.
18% also had Tourette's
14% also had OCD

Primary diagnosis ADD
86% also had dyspraxia
44% had dyslexia
32% had ADHD
20% also had OCD
18% also had Tourette's

Primary diagnosis OCD
84% also had dyspraxia
70% also had ADD

45% also had dyslexia
25% also had ADHD
10% also had Tourette's

Primary diagnosis Tourette's
80% also had ADD
80% also had dyspraxia
38% also had ADHD
24% also had dyslexia
12% also had OCD

It is interesting to note that dyspraxia appears as a prominent symptom in association with each of the primary 'conditions' and that no case of dyslexia, dyspraxia, ADD, ADHD, OCD or Tourette's syndrome was found on its own. In fact the results for finding both Tourette's syndrome and OCD together are perhaps artificially lower than would be expected due to the much lower incidence of these 'conditions' in the general population and therefore also in the study.

Each primary symptom of developmental delay (dyslexia, dyspraxia or whatever) carries with it a variety of potential difficulties for the sufferer. For instance, being dyslexic and/or having attention deficit might well impact severely on your education, which in turn might limit your choice of employment, which may in turn severely reduce your income. Some of the outcomes for sufferers are fairly obvious in terms of employment, etc., but others are not nearly so apparent, for example bullying. Bullying in childhood can have an impact on your personality that lasts a lifetime.

Primary dyslexia

Primary dyslexia is commonly found along with dyspraxia (84 per cent of the time) and attention deficit (62 per cent of the time). Struggling to grasp the basics of reading and constantly failing spelling tests does little to boost your confidence and therefore many children suffer from very low levels of self-esteem. Unless the situation is resolved in childhood, this can have a very damaging effect upon the adolescent as he or she attempts to form meaningful relationships, and can plague a person throughout their life. The child that appears to be not too bright, perhaps wears glasses and constantly drops the ball or falls over can become a laughing stock and a target for bullies.

BULLYING

Bullying is not just something that happens in school. The effects of school bullying can be with you for ever, but if you appear weak you can be bullied in the workplace and in the home. It has been estimated that as many as one person in ten suffers some form of bullying in the workplace, often leading to high levels of absenteeism and serious mental-health issues. There is a fine line between being bullied and being mentally and/or physically abused and it is not just women who suffer.

In childhood the signs of bullying can include becoming withdrawn, crying themselves to sleep, not wanting to go to school, starting to stammer or becoming rude, disobedient, aggressive or bullying younger children. Bullying that takes place during adolescence can lead to depression, anxiety or violent behaviour. Teenage girls are more likely to become aggressive when provoked, while boys are more likely to turn to drink.

School leavers

Leaving school means either starting higher education – college or university – or starting work. Either path marks the start of the passage into adulthood. Without the basic skills of reading, writing and maths the transition from the cosseted school environment into the hard reality of the real world can be tough.

Some people will not only survive the transition but will thrive regardless of how many GCSEs they have. My first employer when I was a boy, working in the summer holidays, could neither read nor write but he made a fortune and was a wonderful human being to boot. Although it is far easier to treat children with learning disabilities than adults, for all the adults out there still struggling to read it is not too late.

Secondary dyslexia

Before moving on, we should consider secondary dyslexia.

It can cause a person great problems, but is also something that can be identified in minutes and treated in weeks.

In order to be able to do any close work – reading, maths, writing, handicrafts, etc. – it is essential that you can bring your eyes in towards the nose so they are both pointing at what you want to look at and, importantly, keep them pointing there. This is known as 'convergence'. Of the children tested at the clinic, 57 per cent had one of the following problems:

1) The eyes could not lock on to the target
2) One eye – usually the left – came in momentarily and then moved out
3) One eye was slow and inaccurate in locking on

Problems locking on to the target are fortunately not that common and are usually found in children with autistic traits. However, if we say that just 50 per cent of the children tested could not converge accurately, then that could equate to 10 per cent of the total adult population having similar problems.

Eye tests
Unfortunately, at the moment very few opticians test for convergence failure and only a few treatment centres exist. However, with 'people power' we can create a demand. If more and more people ask for convergence testing, opticians will build the test into the standard eye exam. I will describe the standard tests for convergence failure and the simple yet highly effective treatment that is available later, but for now ask yourself the following questions in this close-work questionnaire:

1) Did you struggle to learn to read?
2) Do you now read slowly?
3) Do your eyes feel tired or hurt when you are reading?
4) Do you ever see double?
5) Do the words ever move on the page?
6) Does your mind wander when you are reading?
7) Do you sometimes find you have read the same thing twice?
8) Do you get blurred vision?
9) Do you have to keep a finger on the page?
10) Do you dread reading out loud?

If a majority of the answers to the close-work questionnaire were 'Yes' then you might want to try the simple tests described later and think about having a full convergence test carried out.

Primary diagnosis dyspraxia

No matter how old you are, you should not need to suffer the embarrassment of being awkward, uncoordinated and clumsy, or an accident waiting to happen. Developmental dyspraxia is treatable and whether it is because you are tired of constantly knocking things over or you just want to be able to enjoy a game of tennis, it is something you can achieve. Of all the various aspects of developmental delay, developmental dyspraxia has to be the easiest to remedy.

Primary diagnosis Tourette's syndrome

Unlike dyslexia, the signs of Tourette's can be seen, so it is very easy to overlook the less obvious aspects of the developmental delay. Earlier we saw that together with the Tourette's a sufferer is likely to have attention deficit, aspects of hyperactivity, primary and/or secondary dyslexia and almost certainly dyspraxia. As most people with Tourette's use up a huge amount of mental energy trying to suppress the tics, it is hardly surprising that this – on top of all the other signs and symptoms – may severely hinder a person's ability to learn. No matter how bright you are, if you are struggling to learn in the first place and constantly distracted by attention deficit and tics, you are not going to achieve your full potential.

Primary ADD or ADHD

If a child has attention deficit as their most obvious symptom there is a one-in-three chance that they will also be dyslexic, a one-in-six chance of them suffering from OCD or Tourette's and an almost certainty that they will have dyspraxia.

Oppositional Defiance Disorder (ODD)

ODD can follow on from or run in parallel with any of the learning/behavioural disabilities and is characterised by increasing disobedience and 'oppositional behaviour' towards adults, though the child or teenager does not break the law as such.

Although appearing tough on the outside, the youngster is clearly hurting inside. Before puberty it is mainly boys who become oppositional, while after puberty girls can become equally defiant.

ODD INDICATORS

To be considered ODD, five of the eight criteria must be ticked and the behaviour must be present for at least six months.

1) Often loses their temper
2) Often argues with parents/teachers
3) Often openly defiant
4) Often deliberately annoying
5) Often blames others for things that go wrong
6) Often angry and easily annoyed
7) Often spiteful
8) Often swears

Conduct Disorder

A conduct disorder can be thought of as an extension of ODD but includes behaviour and acts that do break the law. Such behaviour may include physical aggression, arson and theft. The early use of tobacco, alcohol and drugs is not uncommon and these young people may also be sexually promiscuous.

Every cloud . . .

Well, perhaps not every cloud, but I am sure on the right day at the right time there is a spark of good in the darkest souls and that spark can be kindled to bring both light and hope to a great many people. Ideally we should be treating children when the first signs of things going wrong become apparent, but adolescents and adults are not beyond help if they want it.

Primary diagnosis OCD

As we will see in Matthew's case history at the end of this chapter, OCD does not occur in isolation and the other symptoms (such as attention deficit in his particular case), can be a huge obstacle to learning. OCD in itself can be very intrusive, occupying ever-increasing periods of time in which rituals have to be performed and, if interrupted or performed incorrectly, repeated again and again until perfected. In childhood the need to perform rituals, either physical or mental, will impact upon learning but, as with Tourette's, there is a hidden side to the 'condition' which is sometimes only seen by the family of the sufferer. The mental energy that it takes to suppress tics or rituals can lead to exhaustion and, like holding your breath, there comes a point when you have to let it out. Unlike holding your breath, which is met with great relief when you finally let it out and breathe in, giving in to a tic or ritual is accompanied by feelings of guilt or failure and this often manifests itself as anger or emotional meltdown.

THE BIG PICTURE

Rather than dealing with the impact of each individual symptom of developmental delay on the adult life of a sufferer in any further detail, it is perhaps more helpful to look at the bigger picture. Regardless of how intelligent you are, both the learning and behavioural aspects of developmental delay will impact upon your education and, if left untreated, will influence your personal profile – your personality.

There are different types of intelligence.

You might be:

- Brilliant at figures but dreadful at spelling
- Good at reading but hopeless at maths or physics
- Amazing at making things with your hands but slow to read
- A genius, but have no common sense whatsoever

Income

It would be very wrong to judge anyone on their academic achievements alone, but the reality of life in the real world is that in terms of income the 'mental powered' jobs tend to be better paid than the manual jobs. Money isn't everything, but in terms of lifestyle it alone decides the house you live in, the car you can afford to buy and run and the number of holidays you take and where you take them (if you get one at all).

Income is also very much related to status. Status is very important to some people; let's face it, we all want to feel important, special, at some point in our lives and if you feel you don't earn enough and haven't achieved enough, it may be hard to feel good about yourself.

Relationships

If your childhood was blighted or you were marginalised by a learning/behavioural problem, your level of confidence might have been severely dented. The passage into adulthood via the often-turbulent adolescent years can be a trying time and if you don't believe in yourself, and can't make friends (particularly with the opposite sex), things can be difficult to say the least.

There is a biological drive in most people to be with others, set up a home and have children. Put simply, the urge to reproduce may appear to be pleasure-driven, but unknowingly we are being enticed to achieve genetic immortality. In other words, if you have children your genes are passed on, and with each succeeding generation your genes continue to survive. But if you lack the confidence to enter into a long-term relationship, it can cause inner conflict; the biological urge is ever present but remains unsatisfied.

You always hurt the one you love

Establishing a relationship can be very difficult for an adult sufferer, and maintaining it even harder. It takes a very special person to live with and cope with the turmoil that is going on in the mind of a sufferer, particularly when the frustrations it generates boil over. A sufferer can wash their hands until they bleed, and mental rituals can become so complex and time-consuming that they occupy the entire day and may even prevent sleep.

Alcoholism, drug abuse and crime

ADHD has been said to be in the region of 10 per cent more common among adults with an alcohol-use disorder than in the general population. In one study it was reported that nearly half of the adults who reported ADHD symptoms also had a substance-abuse disorder (i.e. alcohol or drugs). Earlier, when we considered oppositional defiance disorder it was stated that it can be the forerunner to a conduct disorder, and that this latter condition often goes hand in hand with substance abuse and crime. Developmental delay tends to occur more in boys, as does oppositional defiance disorder, and therefore it isn't surprising to find conduct disorders mainly occurring in boys. We also saw that turning to alcohol as a means of coping is far more common in males.

ADHD is said to be more common in boys although some researchers now say that it may be under-diagnosed in girls. Be that as it may, one thing we do know is that many children are sugar addicts and this is especially true of boys and in particular boys who have been diagnosed as suffering from ADHD.

We will look further at this problem in the next chapter, but for now it is important to realise that it is not all doom and gloom and that regardless of how old you are, help is at hand. DNA is no longer your destiny; with the right advice and a little bit of determination a great many people can change their personal profile and their future.

Case History
My Life with Dyslexia: Matthew Evans

The Early Years

I was born on 1 July 1988. From what I remember, I was completely 'normal' as a young child. I reached milestones early, sitting at three months, crawling by six months and walking unaided at nine months. My journey of struggles started when I started full-time school at the age of four years. I had already attended a nursery school every morning for a year, as is the custom in Wales. School started well, when all that was required was to draw and play, but when the formal learning process began and I was expected to read and write, I was unhappy. This soon developed into a fear of attending school, which would stay with me into later life.

I was lucky to have a teacher in my reception class who was one of only two in the whole of my education to date to make me happy. She was the foundation of getting me through my school life. She was always there for me and she made me feel secure in my own skin.

From the age of about six years, I have had OCD. I would not use the school toilets for fear of catching germs from others, or passing on my germs to them. I would wash my hands profusely, always making sure they were as clean as possible. I could not eat anything that someone else had touched or prepared or if the food had touched another surface that might not be clean. I could not drink a drink if someone had taken a sip from it. This all contributed to a difficult time in school.

At this time, nobody had considered dyslexia. My teacher noticed, when I was five, that I was having difficulty focusing on the words as

I was reading and asked my mum to arrange an eye test, but my eyesight was fine. Then, at age eleven, my mum was concerned when I did not attain a Level 4 in the SATs test, when she knew that I should have. The school was shocked by my result also. When she and my head teacher looked at my paper, I had only managed to complete a third of it. This began to ring alarm bells.

Secondary School

This is when my troubles really started. There were a lot more people around me, which made me very uneasy and self-conscious. Classes gradually got harder in terms of content, which started to really make things worse. I also found it hard to interact with fellow students, as I felt stupid and scared that they would judge me. This was because in class I didn't excel. I had very poor awareness of time and would constantly hand homework in late or leave it until the last minute, putting pressure on myself. I never finished an exam paper and almost always got low marks, which killed any self-confidence I had. My memory was virtually nonexistent, so I could never remember anything I was told. This often got me in trouble, as people thought I was either being silly or just stupid. That isn't to say that I didn't try in the classroom, but I always held back from answering because I thought I was bound to be wrong. This, combined with slow pace and incomplete work, gave teachers a misconception of me as a student. I do admit that sometimes I acted as the class clown, to hide behind the struggle that I faced with schoolwork.

By this time, my mother had trained as a dyslexia teacher and tested me. The results showed that I was dyslexic. My reading and spelling scores were not too bad, but it was speed of information processing, memory and speed of reading and writing that were causing me problems at school. No wonder I never completed class work or exams.

By now, I was also having great trouble with upward motion and would fall over at the top of escalators or getting out of lifts. This led to me having to find alternative ways to get above ground level anywhere, adding to my OCD problems. I developed a huge fear of flying, to the extent that I will not fly independently and avoid it wherever possible. Patterned carpets and wallpaper made me dizzy and these difficulties also affected my social life, leading to me withdrawing socially.

When I was in my final two years of secondary school (Years 10 and 11) and the work was leading to GCSEs, I found myself in the hardest time of my life. I felt sick every single day and it was a regular occurrence for me to be sent home ill, only for me to feel better when I was away from school. Classes were getting too hard for me now. Although school was aware that I had dyslexia, it didn't seem to have registered with any staff and comments like 'Check your work through for spelling errors!' were written in my books. Don't teachers understand that dyslexics don't recognise spelling errors! It was because I was not a severe dyslexic and did not receive Special Educational Needs support that I was ignored. This just added to my frustration. I would get very angry because people did not understand my perspective of things.

Classes were getting too much for me now. In maths, I was a top-set student, but when quick-fire questions were asked, I froze. I couldn't work out answers quickly on the spot. All the other students would get the answer way before me and this made me feel like the most stupid person alive. In English lessons, my rate of writing was considerably slower than anyone else's and my reading was slow and monotone. In French, I had a good understanding, but when it came to remembering words, I just couldn't do it. As for science, I understood everything, but couldn't put this into practice.

By now my self-esteem was rock bottom and I was so self-conscious that my social life was affected to the extent that I could not go out with friends. If I did venture out to a disco, I usually left early because the flashing lights made me feel dizzy, faint and nauseous. This time in my life was very low. I wasn't doing well at school and my social life was nonexistent. This was the first time in my life that I considered suicide. I was so unhappy, I just couldn't deal with my life any more.

At about this time I saw a behavioural optometrist, who tested the behaviour of my eyes. He found that they were not working together at all and arranged for me to have coloured lenses. I struggled through my GCSEs and with the help of the tinted lenses I actually finished an English exam for the first time ever (and passed).

Further Education College

I moved on to college where, at a time so low in my life, I met the second teacher who made me feel comfortable and able. He understood that I was struggling and helped me out. He surpassed his job description with me and, with his help, I came to enjoy going to college to *learn and work. He pushed me, to make me see that I could do things – and do them well. He was always there for me and made my self-confidence rise and for that I am very thankful. Without him to guide me at this time I would have probably dropped out of college and not be where I am now. I studied Sports Science, as I wanted to become a professional sportsman. The funny thing is that even though my eyes do not work together, I am a good golfer and a fast bowler in cricket. When asked how I managed to take wickets, I had to admit that I close my eyes at the last minute, as I can't focus on the stumps because they blur! If only the batsmen facing me knew that!*

I am now able to embrace the fact that I have dyslexia. With the help of Dr Pauc, my life is great. I feel 'cured' of dyslexia and have very few of my previous problems to deal with. When I first went to see Dr Pauc, I was feeling very low, having dropped out of university and so missing the chance of training with a county cricket team. His treatment has given me a new lease of life and the confidence to move forward. For that I am very grateful.

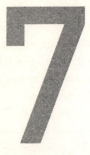

THE IMPACT UPON SOCIETY OF LEARNING AND BEHAVIOURAL PROBLEMS

It is undeniable that learning and behavioural problems have an impact on society. But we must also consider if society best serves those amongst us that suffer from these 'conditions'.

THE EFFECT ON LITERACY

Wikipedia definition of literacy:

The traditional definition of literacy is considered to be the ability to read and write, or the ability to use language to read, write, listen, and speak. In modern contexts, the word refers to reading and writing at a level adequate for communication, or at a level that lets one understand and communicate ideas in a literate society, so as to take part in that society.

The last part of this definition really gets at the hub of the problem, as it is not just the inability to read and write that is so important but the fact that if you can't communicate properly, you are effectively unable to participate fully in the society in which you live. If you cannot read, this could mean you have a smaller vocabulary, and this may limit your comprehension of the spoken word.

Functional literacy

But it's not just a case of being *able* to read – you have to be able to use what you've read. The Organisation for Economic Co-operation and Development defines functional literacy not as the ability to read and write but as 'whether a person is able to understand and employ printed information in daily life, at home, at work and in the community'.

Being illiterate can make you a stranger in your own land and without help you cannot escape this alienation. Similarly, if you struggle to read and therefore do not find it enjoyable, your vocabulary is less likely to build and your knowledge base will be restricted to that which you can gain via the spoken word. A survey conducted in 2000 reported that a large proportion of adults in the UK have serious literacy problems and found that in the multi-nation study the UK was fourteenth out of twenty in a list charting the percentage of adults who read a book at least once a month.

Case History: Harry Carpenter

Harry was my first adult patient who approached me specifically for help with his dyslexia. At our first meeting he told me how he had struggled at school, had received numerous cuffs about the ear for being lazy, and was eventually told he was thick and placed with all the other boys that would never do well, to be taught gardening, metalwork and woodwork. It was this last activity that was to prove to be the one thing he excelled at and the only subject in the whole curriculum that he truly understood.

Leaving school he was fortunate enough to get an apprenticeship with a very good firm of carpenters and joiners. Because of his natural ability and his love of wood, his work was always good and because he was shown everything he needed to know he had no problem in learning his trade. However, several times during his career he was offered the position of foreman, but every time he turned it down even though it meant he would forego the increase in wages associated with the promotion. Harry knew that without reading and writing he would not be able to cope as a foreman and so had to turn down this betterment to his career.

Harry had married shortly after completing his apprenticeship and throughout their married life it was his wife who had dealt with

*the post, getting insurance, organising holidays, etc. At the age of 64
and with retirement looming it was only now that Harry had decided
that he would really like to learn to read.*

BELIEVE IT OR NOT

- Eight million people in the UK are said to be so poor at reading and writing that they cannot cope with the demands of modern life.
- 10 per cent of the UK population were unable to read the instructions on a packet of seeds.
- 29 per cent of the UK adult population could not calculate the area of a floor either in square feet or metres.
- Less than one third of the adult population could work out the amount of liner required to line a pond even when provided with a calculator, pen and paper.
- 40 per cent of adults in some parts of England cannot read or write adequately nor carry out simple additions.
- 24 per cent of the UK population are functionally illiterate and this figure rises to 40 per cent in some regions.
- 12 per cent of young adults admitted to having problems with reading, writing, spelling and basic maths.
- 30 per cent of adults believe their skills do not meet the demands of the 'information age'.

The statistics above were taken from various surveys conducted between 1998 and 2005, and the figures are likely to be getting worse. We know that all the manifestations of learning and behavioural disorders in children are increasing at a frightening rate; clearly if this is not properly addressed we are going to find that the problem of adult literacy can only worsen as these children become adults.

Counting the cost of behaviour and learning difficulties

The cost of caring for a person with autism has been estimated to be approximately £20,000 per year. Special Educational Needs funding has risen by more than £1 billion since 2002–3 to £4.5 billion in 2006–7. In addition to this some parents spend up to £10,000 per year to provide private tutoring and/or treatment for their children. For those parents who opt for a private education for their child, working on the basis that smaller class sizes and greater SEN provision will help their child, the cost can be several thousand pounds per term.

There are also hidden costs to society, as we must not forget the human suffering that so often accompanies these 'conditions'. One survey found that two out of three employees who failed to show up for work weren't actually physically ill but cited family issues (21 per cent), personal needs (18 per cent), and stress (12 per cent) for unscheduled absences. Stress itself may be brought on by any number of factors, but bullying in the workplace was cited as being a major factor and there has been a rise in the number of bullying cases reported to unions and workplace helplines in recent years.

THE CONFEDERATION OF BRITISH INDUSTRY (CBI) ANNUAL REPORT 2006 REVEALED:

- Absences increased in 2006 as workers took an average of seven days off sick
- This is calculated to have resulted in a total of 175 million lost working days
- This cost the economy an incredible £13.4 billion
- 72 per cent of long-term absences in non-manual jobs are caused by stress

---

ALCOHOLISM

We have already looked at the link between ADHD and substance abuse in adolescence and adulthood. It has been suggested that as many as one in ten teenagers and adults have problems associated with alcohol consumption, with one study stating that the probability of alcohol abuse in ADHD sufferers may be three and a half times greater than that of the general population. Clearly not everyone that has a problem with the demon drink will have suffered some form of developmental delay as a child, but we have seen already how a great many people who have suffered bullying as a result of, say, dyspraxia have resorted to drink and the increased likelihood in those people with a history of ADHD. Those that do have this problem run the risk of trouble with the law and/or the need for medical attention. In the long term, alcohol abuse can lead to the break-up of the family unit and personal ruin.

The cost of alcoholism
The cost to the UK (in 2003) was £7.3 billion per annum to fund policing, prevention services and processing individuals through the courts.

ALCOHOL AND CRIME

At the time of their arrest . . .

- 50 per cent of people arrested for breach of the peace
- 45 per cent arrested for criminal damage
- 30 per cent of those arrested for burglary

. . . tested positive for alcohol.

CRIME AND PUNISHMENT

Most individuals with learning and behavioural difficulties will never commit a serious crime. However, of those in trouble with the law you might expect that many have some form of behavioural or learning difficulty. The results of some studies of juvenile offenders would suggest that as many as 70 per cent have ADHD. It has been suggested that up to 40 per cent of male prisoners in medium-risk facilities have the classic symptoms of ADHD; when you consider that in the general population the occurrence of ADHD is in the region of 5 per cent, this is a very worrying figure. If these figures are accurate then we have to ask ourselves who is the real culprit and why is it that these prisoners are being punished and not treated?

It is my belief and that of a great many serious scientists that there is a very real link between food additives and behavioural problems – and especially in the case of ADHD sufferers (see also Chapter 10). Perhaps we should be looking elsewhere for the real villains and providing treatment for the unwitting victims of their crimes.

> Some campaigners have argued that crime could be halved in as little as ten years if ADHD was addressed and treated.

SOLVING THE PROBLEM

It's important not to get bogged down in doom and gloom. Instead we really need to look at just what we can do to remedy the situation.

Secondary dyslexia (the inability to bring the eyes in towards the nose before you can read efficiently) is easily treated but must be accurately assessed first (see Chapter 6), and more opticians would offer this test if there were greater awareness of and demand for it.

The provisions of the Disability Discrimination Act 1995 (UK) cover people who have difficulties carrying out normal everyday activities, on a long-term basis, as a result of a physical or mental impairment. Being dyslexic or dyspraxic can cause all sorts of problems in the workplace, from other people not being able to read your writing to struggling to keep pace with a production line. Under the terms of the Act, employers must ensure that their employees with dyspraxia, dyslexia, etc., are given appropriate support to minimise the impact of their symptoms so they can not only cope but hopefully thrive in the workplace.

The stuff of life

Dealing with the impact of developmental delay is all very well and is to be commended, but wouldn't it be better to address the cause of this ever-increasing problem and then do everything we can to keep us all functioning at the highest possible level? In the past the government has stepped in to address problems facing the nation with measures such as the introduction of milk in schools and school dinners. Is it now not the time for the government to act again?

Just as milk was introduced into schools in 1946, why not now provide every child in school with a daily dose of the omega-3s that have been proven to be so important for brain function (see Chapter 10)? The beneficial effects of omega-3 are well known, as is the fact that it is lacking in the diet of the vast majority of both children and adults. We have all read about the various trials that have been carried out in schools or have watched TV documentaries that have shown how children taking omega-3 are calmer, more attentive and achieve better SAT results.

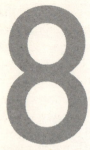

ASSESSING THE ADULT WITH DEVELOPMENTAL DELAY SYNDROME

TAKING A HISTORY

In terms of understanding a person, their individual history is the key. If you really want to understand the thinking behind a great philosopher's ideas or the motivation behind a writer's work, you need to read their biography. Philosophers and writers are only human and everything from a physical disability to the politics of the age when they lived will colour how they see the world. Similarly, to truly understand someone sitting in front of you, you need to know not just their own history but the history of their family as well.

When I take the history of a child the situation is usually very straightforward; as at least one parent will be sitting in front of me and the chances are that one or more grandparents are still alive and can fill in any gaps that the parent can't remember. However, with an adult patient things can be very different and often big gaps are missing in the developmental history, which requires a bit of research to fill or may indeed remain missing. When taking a child's history it is possible to learn a lot about the family set-up, socioeconomic status and history just by observing the parents.

The starting point when taking down a case history (and no more is this true than with the learning/behavioural disabilities) is the family history. Because there is such an overlap in symptoms in every individual patient and the link between family members is so strong, it is essential to tease out as much information as possible. This may require a little bit of research on the part of the adult sufferer but is well worth attempting. Without this kind of information, for example if the person was adopted, there is no choice but to start with whatever information can be gleaned purely from the patient.

Ideally, the personal history should start as far back as when their mother was pregnant, as we know that such things as maternal stress can have an influence on developmental delay, as can premature birth. Then we need details of the birth including the length of labour, method of delivery and whether there was any 'foetal distress' during the birth. As all human offspring are born 'prematurely' (see Chapter 1) – while the brain is still developing at an embryonic growth rate – a birth at less than 38 weeks or a difficult birth can make someone more likely to suffer a developmental delay and later learning and/or behavioural difficulties.

Factors during birth that raise the probability of development delay

- Maternal illness or stress
- Primary foetal distress e.g. getting stuck in the birth canal or having the umbilical cord wrapped around the neck
- Secondary foetal distress – assisted delivery by forceps/ventouse
- Trauma
  - dislocation or fracture, e.g. broken collar bone
  - haemorrhage, e.g. bleeding under the scalp or inside the skull

Once we know how the baby was delivered it is necessary to know whether he or she was healthy, breast- or bottle-fed and whether or not there were any feeding problems. Then it is essential to record as many of the developmental milestones as possible. The milestones provide a pretty good idea as to how the nervous system is developing generally but also gives some pretty good clues as to how the various regions of the brain are maturing. Humans walk on two legs, so the stages in the transition from crawling on all fours to walking upright – literally defying gravity – are of huge importance. We also have and use other faculties and abilities that are unique. The two-legged posture and freeing up the hands for purposes other than crawling has allowed us to develop manual dexterity and this extensive skilled use of the hands has been said to have led to the evolution – expansion and development – of the human brain.

OUR UNIQUE ABILITIES

- We are 'obligate bipeds' – we walk on our hind legs
- Manual dexterity – we use our hands for fine motor skills
- Tools – we make and use tools so we can do more with our hands
- Speech – we use highly sophisticated speech
- Writing – we use our hands to produce writing to communicate
- Painting – we produce works of art
- Stereoscopic vision – both eyes face forward and look at the same target
- Reading – we produce books to inform and entertain
- Mathematics – we use numbers
- Music – we sing and play instruments
- Teach – we provide formal education
- Dress – we wear clothes
- Continence – we learn to control our bladder
- Time – we use timepieces and can think in time
- Thoughts – we can imagine and communicate these imaginings
- Invent – we can create new ideas and objects
- Cooking – we prepare and cook food

Crawling, standing and walking

If at all possible it is very useful to know when the child first sat, if they crawled and when they started walking. These motor (movement) developmental stages give the practitioner vital clues to when movement programmes and muscle tone were established. Crawling is said to be critical in the development of collections of nerve cells in the spinal cord that, when stimulated, generate the repetitive, rhythmic movements needed for walking, swimming, etc. These developmental stages are often delayed in association with learning/behavioural difficulties but as in the case of Matthew, can occur too soon.

A wee achievement

The next thing we need to know is when bladder control was attained, firstly by day and then by night. We all expect babies to be in nappies but at around two to two and a half years we expect to see sufficient bladder control – with a few accidents – for the nappy to be done away with during the day and shortly afterwards also at night. Continued wetting by day is not a good sign. Staying dry through the night can often take longer to achieve and some children, usually boys, may take several years to become reliably continent at night. The importance of bladder control lies in the fact that the micturition centre – the executive centre for bladder control – is situated in the brain's frontal cortex. This means that continence gives a measure of how well this very important area of the brain is developing.

Learning to speak

The next very important step to consider is the development of speech. Generally speaking – no pun intended – in the first year there should be a collection of simple words in place, followed in the second year by the use of two words together – 'me come, you go' – leading on to mini-sentences in the third year. Minor speech delays are not uncommon but should always be taken into consideration. Major speech delays are a real concern and will be picked up during the standard developmental assessments and if necessary referred on to speech therapy.

Social skills and academic progress

Going to a nursery is often the first big step towards honing your social skills. It is a chance to mix with other children, often for the first time without having your mother close at hand for moral support and guidance. Learning to play with other children – sharing, cooperating, etc. – allows children to develop the basic skills necessary to exist within the tight restraints of a complex modern society. It is also a time when any problems in this area of development should be picked up. The child that fails to integrate, plays at the edges of the group, does not talk, may be just very shy but similarly may be showing signs of autistic traits. Children who are boisterous, unable to sit still and show impulsive behaviour may already be heading towards ADHD. Aggressive behaviour may be the result of a child being too full-on, lacking restraint or may indicate that there are troubles brewing.

Some nursery schools incorporate a little formal learning into the day, but once into reception classes the business of learning begins in earnest. It is at this stage that difficulties in reading may be picked up which, if undiagnosed and consequently not treated, can plague an individual for a lifetime. As we have seen already (and will go on to describe in some detail later) secondary dyslexia is so easy to diagnose and equally easy to treat, and this diagnosis makes learning so much easier and prevents so much misery. Although problems with learning to read often run in parallel with problems in learning to spell, it does not always follow that the child will struggle with maths, and this shows that their brains are basically fine.

Learning to write

Poor handwriting and indeed how you hold the pencil or pen is another problem that is often found in association with dyslexia – and again something that can end up being a real pain, literally. How and why we hold a pencil the way we do is a little complicated to explain but also something that a lot of professionals understand only poorly. In order to have a relaxed comfortable grip it is necessary to have the correct tone in the muscles of the hand and the second-generation neurons (see Chapter 1) need to be working as they should.

Setting the muscle tone for each side of the body is a major function of the brain's cerebellum. Each hemisphere (side) of the brain sets the tone for its side of the body but it does this generally rather than specifically for individual muscles. Now here we have a problem because we use more muscles to bend the arm than to straighten it. So, if the more powerful muscles aren't toned down, the arm will be held in a position that resembles that of somebody who has had a stroke. To stop this, the brain has to send messages down to the more powerful muscles, basically reducing the amount of tone, so that you can write without your arm being held permanently bent. However, you also need to be able to produce fine, controlled movements of the fingers and wrist so that you can produce good handwriting, and this is one of the functions of the dark side of the brain.

Checking the wiring

Most people are right-handed and in theory should also be right-footed and have a dominant right eye. However, this is not always the case and some people will be left-handed or may have mixed handedness when they're doing different things. To check for the dominant eye, I simply hand a telescope to the patient and ask them to look out of the window. Checking for the dominant ear is not so easy as people tend to get into the habit of using a particular ear, which is more to do with ease rather than dominance.

Where did things start?

In an ideal world it would be possible to find out exactly when things started to go wrong and who picked up on it. With children this generally isn't difficult but with adult patients it can prove to be a real problem. As the vast majority (and I would say all) of the symptoms of developmental delay are said to start in childhood then knowing what, when and how bad they were helps to build a detailed picture of the individual's problems. This may require a little research but is a very worthwhile exercise. If the parents are no longer alive, then an aunt or older brother or sister might be able to fill in some of the missing details.

Learning about dyspraxia

In order to gain some insight into dyspraxic tendencies, it's often necessary to ask certain questions that are designed to bring out further information. For instance, asking about learning to dress yourself can lead on to such things as sequencing skills. Some children simply struggle to fit all those toes into a sock, while others not only struggle to accomplish the task but also cannot work out the order in which the clothes need to be put on and, rather like Superman, can end up with their underwear on top of their trousers.

Although there are various tests that can be carried out later during the examination that will provide very good indications of how the brain and cerebellum (a region of the brain) are functioning, a huge amount of information can be gained from the developmental history and by simply observing the person from the moment they enter the clinic.

DYSPRAXIC TENDENCY QUESTIONS

1) Did you struggle to learn to dress yourself?
2) Were you a messy eater?

---

3) Were you accident-prone?
4) Did you make frequent visits to your hospital's Accident &
Emergency department?
5) Were you clumsy?
6) Were you late to learn to ride a bike?
7) Did you struggle to catch a ball?
8) Did you hate sports?
9) Did you bump into things and/or knock things over?
10) Was your handwriting poor?

More answers with 'Yes' equals a greater probability of dyspraxia

Case History: Paddy T, age 24

I came to Tinsley House Clinic having always known that I had poten-
tial that was being held back in some way, and this stemmed from an
annoying childhood inability to play ball sports – most notably foot-
ball, cricket, rugby, tennis and volleyball – despite being active and
healthy. The teasing was regular but I was a popular child and was
able to laugh it off and come up with strategies to avoid looking too
inept. In the end I took up rowing, where I was able to succeed. I was
bright, but always disorganised and poor at time management. I
would also easily switch off if what I was trying to learn didn't seem
directly relevant at the time. I enjoyed the structure in the school system
and this allowed me to do well at my schoolwork despite my problems.

However, at university I was unable to take charge of self-directed
learning and severely underperformed in my degree. I still got value
from the rowing team at university because the team and coaches pro-
vided the structure that I needed to do well, just like at school. Reading
had always been a problem, and despite being a capable reader I could
never do it for pleasure, excepting the odd interesting magazine article.

As far as most people were concerned I was competitive, lazy and
slightly uncoordinated. To quote a friend, I was bad at 'stuff'.

Since starting at Tinsley House in March 07 I have noticed a huge
improvement in my ball skills. Before it would be hit and miss if I caught
an object, now it is more predictable and the outcome doesn't take me by
surprise. This was most noticeable during a game of beach volleyball
when some friends pointed out that I was considerably better than in

games we had played the previous year, almost a new player! I was very happy to hear this. I no longer have to laugh off being incapable.

Otherwise changes have been significant but less noticeable. I feel more at home and confident in a busy crowded room. I find reading easier, the words are easier to 'follow' on the page and my eyes feel more relaxed, although I still haven't been able to read for pleasure. Time management is still an issue but I feel that I am on the right track. I look forward to what will come next. The changes have not been in a logical order, and some things have happened in a more subtle way than others. Despite being a mild case, I am increasingly feeling more normal, like the person I am meant to be, rather than an ambitious struggling fool who doesn't know why he is bad at stuff.

Short-term memory

All children are said to have a poor short-term memory, and this is something a lot of adults have problems with, too. But is it truly a matter of memory or could it simply be that they are not listening? Most ladies realise there is little point in discussing such important things as the purchase of a new handbag while their partner is trying to get the football results off the TV. It just isn't going to work, and the reason why is focus.

Children and adults with attention deficit do not necessarily have a poor short-term memory. Instead they struggle to keep what is often mundane (to them) information in their memory and this is frequently made worse by them being very easily distracted. It is very important to differentiate between these two functions and provide a test of short-term memory during the consultation process.

SHORT-TERM MEMORY TEST

1) Read the following list of items to yourself
2) Read it again out loud
3) Say it again – but in a whisper

The items are:

a) A piece of wood
b) A snail shell
c) A piece of seaweed

See if you can remember these three items by the time you have finished this chapter.

Routines are nice, rituals are not

Many people can be creatures of habit, preferring to stick to their own little routines, and this type of behaviour can be mistaken for rituals. Indeed, there is a very fine line between routines and rituals, particularly in childhood, but it is essential to be able to separate the two when taking a detailed case history. Routines can be a comfort and if the right side of the brain is not functioning as it should then avoiding new situations also avoids the stress that often accompanies them. Minor obsessive traits are very common in childhood and can be carried over into adult life.

However, this is very different from the rituals of OCD that are not only very time-consuming but also stressful.

Activity levels

Assessing the normal daily level of activity in an adult, particularly during a formal consultation, can be very difficult and often it is necessary to ask relatives or friends to gain an accurate picture. Questions about the level of activity at work, at home and while attending social or sporting events should be asked. If you have an active physical job, your active nature can be lost within the normal processes of the day – but at home you may find it impossible to keep still.

Tics

If a tic disorder forms part of a developmental delay, it is very important to chart its progress through childhood, and note the different types of tics that occur during various stages and phases. It is important to note any progression from minor facial tics (blinking or grimacing) to larger motor tics and perhaps vocal tics (sounds). It's also important to know whether the periods of consistent tics or progressions were related to events in life or particularly stressful times.

Traits

Lastly, before considering the individual's medical history and diet, it is a good idea, if at all possible, to have the answers to the following questions:

1) As a young child did you ever walk on tiptoe?
2) Did you ever flap your hands from the wrist?
3) Did you ever spin yourself or objects on a very regular basis?
4) Did you make good eye contact?
5) Were you affectionate?

Ideally questions 1 to 3 should be 'No' and 4 to 5 should be 'Yes'.

Medical history

Taking a detailed medical history not only helps the practitioner gain a measure of the patient's general health, but it can also reveal vital clues as to their past immune status – their ability to ward off disease. Also, a history of numerous knocks, bangs, falls and crashes can complete an already vivid picture of the early years. A vaccination history plus any medications being taken should complete the history.

Food and diet

I like to keep the questioning about food and drink intake in a structured format, rather than just saying, 'Is your diet OK?' Therefore, I like to know exactly when and what the first thing eaten in the morning is, and to monitor the intake of food, drinks and treats throughout the day until bedtime.

All of the following need to be considered:

● Morning tea/coffee plus breakfast
● Mid-morning snack
● Lunch
● Afternoon tea, tea break, snacks
● Dinner
● Supper
● Drinks during the day including water, tea, coffee, fizzy drinks and alcohol
● Sweets, chocolates, cakes or biscuits consumed or kept in the car or office

Knowing exactly what you are eating and where provides very good clues as to the amount of salt, sugar, trans fats, artificial sweeteners and additives you are expecting your body and brain to cope with.

Testing times

By the time the practitioner gets round to examining you, he or she should have a very good idea of what the situation is; in most cases the tests are really just to confirm the diagnosis. However, although it is the responsibility of the experienced practitioner to carry out the examination, there are certain tests and procedures that you should expect to be carried out.

I will not go into any great detail here but will highlight the various tests that I believe should be carried out and will provide a brief explanation as to why they are needed.

My standard examination includes a physical examination, hearing tests, eye tests and a neurological examination that includes cranial nerve testing, cerebellar tests and peripheral nerve testing. As and when necessary further tests can be carried out or requested.

- **Physical examination** – height, weight, body mass index, blood pressure (both sides), pulse, respiration, etc.
- **Hearing tests** – using tympanography, otoacoustic emission testing, etc.
- **Eye tests** – distance vision, visual fields, pupil responses to light, accommodation, convergence and a quick look into the eyes.
- **Cranial nerves** – these should be assessed in order (there are twelve cranial nerves). The ability to smell and to know what it is you are smelling is very important as this gives a clue as to how well the right frontal cortex is functioning. Also, differences in sensory appreciation should be noted as this provides good clues as to what is happening in the parietal cortex (back of the brain).
- **Cerebellar testing** – at least four tests should be carried out.
- **Peripheral testing** – this should include the arms and legs, and apart from the usual sensory tests should include tests for muscle strength and tone plus the deep and superficial reflexes.
- **Computer-generated tests** – selected and tested as necessary but must include convergence testing.

And finally

By now there should be a complete and detailed history of your personal developmental history that can be related to how the specific areas of your brain function.

Now we simply have to put in place a specific treatment regime designed to address mental health and stimulate the areas of physiological weakness in terms of brain function.

NOW – WHAT WERE THOSE THREE THINGS YOU HAD TO REMEMBER?

IT'S NOT TOO LATE – TREATING THE ADULT WITH DDS

A DRUG-FREE TREATMENT

The first question I have to ask any parent seeking treatment for an older child is 'Will they be compliant?' In other words, there is no point in going through the whole consultation and examination process if the child or teenager is going to refuse to comply with the treatment regime. With adult patients this doesn't apply, as having decided for themselves that they need help, one assumes they will be more than pleased to follow the guidelines. But we must bear in mind that it does require a certain amount of personal discipline and perseverance to be successful.

The treatment regime is divided into four parts, and each must be carried out simultaneously if the package is going to work. There are numerous treatments currently on offer based on dietary change, exercise, psychotherapy, medication, etc., but I believe that if you use any of them alone they will all fall short of the patient's expectations. Although each individual approach has its own particular virtues and may provide some benefit, in isolation they are destined to fail.

I will explain why – if we look at what is currently on offer we will see the shortfalls each treatment approach has.

You are what you eat
Numerous excellent books are now available which will extol the virtues of a healthy diet, explain why you need a balanced diet and will

even provide menu planners and recipes. Unfortunately, unless you are an Inuit it is unlikely that you will be getting enough omega-3 essential fatty acids in your diet and therefore, as the brain needs a good regular supply of omega-3 to be at the peak of fitness, we already have hit a major snag.

A gymnasium for the mind

Also, just like your body, your brain needs regular exercise to stay fit and if it is suffering for any reason, it needs specific carefully regulated exercise to help it on its way.

We are now all familiar with the little electronic gadgets that can be used on a regular basis to exercise the mind. That and doing crossword puzzles are excellent ways of keeping the mind active, but again on their own they are no more than an aid to keeping mentally fit.

There are also expensive treatment programmes based on doing physical exercises aimed at treating dyslexia, dyspraxia, etc. But again, without the right diet, supplementation with omega-3s, vitamins and minerals, together with providing treatments aimed at the areas of brain that are underfunctioning, they may help, but they won't have the impact that is intended.

A FOUR-PRONGED APPROACH – DIET + SUPPLEMENTATION + PHYSICAL EXERCISES + COMPUTER PROGRAM

Diet – food for thought

As any good builder will tell you, if you want to build a house the most important thing is to get the foundations right, and anyone who has suffered from settlement cracks will know exactly what I mean. So it is with the treatment plan, with the diet and supplementation needing to be in place before we can progress on to the computer-generated treatment programmes. The aims of the diet are:

1) To eliminate, as far as possible, bad E numbers from the diet
2) To totally eliminate aspartame from the diet
3) To monitor carbohydrate intake
4) To monitor and limit the amount of trans fats in the diet
5) To monitor salt intake

6) To provide the right foods at the right time
7) To ensure proper hydration

Supplements – what to add

There are some nutrients that, even in a healthy diet, are difficult to get in sufficient amounts, particularly if you are suffering from a developmental delay.

Therefore the treatment programme recommends:

- Essential fatty acids daily – a double dose for three months and a single dose thereafter
- For adults add 15mg zinc sulphate and magnesium daily
- Vitamin B complex
- Vitamin C

You'll find more details of the supplements in Chapter 11.

Now add exercise

General exercise

There is a simple logic to the treatment plan. First deal with the diet, and then add both general and specific exercises. You don't have to join the local gym but you do need to establish a routine to ensure you get regular exercise on a weekly basis. Some people find that the motivation of being a member of a club is helpful in order to make sure that they do exercise at least twice a week, though with several hundred pounds going out of your bank account each year you do need to make sure that you get your money's worth, and if work or family commitments make a twice-weekly visit to the gym impractical, you might think about incorporating some physical exercise into your daily routine. If at all possible walk or use your bike to get to work, go for a swim in your lunch hour and whenever possible use the stairs. Or at the weekend you could take the kids out for a long bike ride.

In order for your exercising to be beneficial you do need to get a little out of puff and to work up something of a sweat. Ambling along at two miles a fortnight is not going to get your heart pumping and the blood whizzing round the body. On the other hand, if you are not used to having regular exercise you will need to take things gently and pace yourself at first or seek advice from a fitness expert.

Brain exercises

Once the dietary advice has been put in place and you understand the need for regular general exercise, you need to establish a daily regime of exercises designed to challenge the brain's cerebellum.

The first exercise is progressive and is designed to challenge the cerebellum on both sides with the intention of bringing the two hemispheres (left and right sides of the cerebellum) into synch – see 1 to 4 below. The second simple exercise that can be built into your daily routine is designed to stimulate the side of the cerebellum that is flagging. You'll learn how to do these exercises in Chapter 13.

1) With your hands by your side, your head in a neutral position and eyes closed, walk up and then down three stairs, three times, three times a day (never go higher than three steps). When you can do three repetitions perfectly, do five, then seven. Once you have mastered forward stair-walking, do it backwards with the same progressions.

2) Once you can stair-walk forwards and backwards, start forward stair-walking again, but this time carrying a tray with a plastic tumbler full of water on it.

3) Each day when brushing your teeth, use your left hand and stand on your left leg. (Do the tests listed below to check which hand and foot to use – usually the left.)

4) Do exercise one until perfect, then two until perfect. Then you should complete exercise three at least twice a day.

Caution – when first starting the progressive stair-walking exercise have a friend or your partner close at hand in case you stumble or fall. This can be discontinued once you have progressed and feel confident to exercise alone.

A balanced mind

Because the different exercises are specific to the left or right side of the cerebellum or brain, if you have not had the benefit of a formal assessment you need to do a few simple tests before starting the initial mini-regime. The tests, along with other exercises that can then be carried out at home, will be described later in the book.

Following an assessment at the clinic, a patient would be sent home with a list of supplements to be taken daily, together with various dietary 'Do's and don'ts' and at least the two simple exercises for the cerebellum, based on the clinical findings. A follow-up appointment would be made for four to six weeks to give the dietary changes and supplementation time to start to have an effect.

At that second assessment the patient would be questioned about how well they had done at implementing the dietary changes and which brand of supplements they were taking. As the amount of omega-3 and -6 varies between the brands and some products contain the artificial sweetener aspartame it is always worth checking which brand is being used. Having gone over the diet and supplements it is necessary to check that the exercises have been carried out on a regular basis, before asking the patient if they have noticed any changes.

The second assessment gives the practitioner an opportunity to re-examine the patient and to compare the results with the previous visit. If you decide to follow the advice given in this book and start your own exercise routine, while following the dietary advice, it is worthwhile doing the set of tests again after six to eight weeks and getting someone to compare the results. There is nothing like being told how much you have improved to give your confidence a real boost and, if you are already feeling the benefit of the diet, it is all you need to motivate you to carry on.

Once you have your diet under control and you have mastered these simple exercises you will be ready for either more advanced physical exercises or the computer-generated programmes described later in the book.

Remember – nothing ventured, nothing gained.

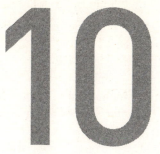

NUTRITION AND THE BRAIN

OUR CHANGING DIETS

The way we eat has changed dramatically over the past thirty or so years – and not for the better. Admittedly, in some respects, our diets have improved: we're drinking more skimmed milk and less full fat; and we eat more wholemeal bread and less white bread. We're also eating less salt, and more fruit. But still, the progress is too little and too slow, with very few people meeting all their dietary targets, such as the maximum for salt, the minimum for fibre, and the five-a-day target for fruit and vegetables.

No longer do we shop on a daily basis, visiting the local shops to purchase fresh food that was wrapped in paper before being handed to us or selected, weighed and placed in a brown paper bag. Eating out was a thing for high days and holidays unless you were rich or famous, and most meals were taken while seated round the dining table.

Many dietary trends have been in the wrong direction. We're eating less vegetables than thirty years ago, more meat products such as burgers and sausages (as opposed to 'real' meat and offal), and we're drinking more fizzy drinks. Also, our purchases of ready-meals have gone through the roof.

Some ready-meals aren't so bad. But you really do need to check the nutritional labelling, as many of them are worryingly high in calories, fat (especially saturated fat), salt and sugar. To increase their shelf life, ready-meals also generally contain artificial preservatives, and often colourings, flavourings and sweeteners to make them more appealing. In addition, the portion sizes are huge compared to those people cooked for themselves thirty years ago.

Go back sixty years, and you'll find people eating 59 per cent more fish and 34 per cent more vegetables than we do today.

We're eating far less fresh, nutritious home-cooked food, while our intake of processed food, high in fat, sugar, salt and additives, has rocketed. Between 1980 and 2000 the amount of food we ate outside the home increased by 40 per cent – and away from our own kitchens we tend to eat more, from menus where we have no control over the ingredients. Our intake of fast food – whose portions are expanding all the time – has also risen.

What our bodies and brains need is a return to good home cooking, using simple wholesome ingredients, and plenty of fresh food. Then, we'd control what goes into our meals, increase our nutrient intake, and we'd remove the need for a lot of artificial additives.

WHAT'S IN IT FOR ME?

You know that a healthy diet is important to keep you feeling strong and fit, and to maintain a healthy weight. You might even know about the effect that diet can have on your risk of conditions and diseases such as high blood pressure, atherosclerosis ('furring' of the arteries), heart disease, stroke, cancer, type-2 diabetes and osteoporosis.

But something that fewer people are aware of is the immense impact that their food has on their brain. Good nutrition is essential for building healthy brains, and keeping them that way.

It's crucial for mothers to eat healthily during their pregnancy, and also when breast-feeding, to provide their babies with the nutrients their developing brains (and bodies) need.

Until fairly recently, it was believed that brain development 'finished' at childhood – any damage after that was irreparable, and after your teenage years, in terms of brain function (if not knowledge and wisdom) it was downhill all the way.

Things have changed, and scientists now know that the brain is remarkably flexible throughout life. It is constantly being remodelled, and new connections made between brain cells. This makes it all the more important to keep the brain well nourished, with all the raw materials it needs for growth and repair, plus quality fuel to keep it firing on all cylinders.

Perhaps the notion of 'brain food' isn't so far-fetched after all. The brain has certain very specific nutritional needs, and by paying attention to these, you can expect to reap the benefits. And the good news is that there's nothing strange or esoteric about these foods – they all have their place in that healthy balanced diet we should be eating in order to live longer, healthier lives. And what's more, they're easy to prepare and tasty as well. Nothing that tastes of cardboard or sawdust.

A 'brain friendly' diet is important in helping support treatment for learning disabilities. It can also help anyone to:

- Improve their ability to concentrate
- Improve and maintain their energy levels
- Stay calm and focused
- Help reduce feelings of frustration/aggression
- Boost their learning ability and intellectual performance
- Improve their memory

CAN DIET 'BOOST' THE BRAIN?

It's undeniable that nutritional deficiencies can lead to psychological symptoms, but can certain foods actually *improve* your brain's performance?

There is little evidence that 'superfoods' or supplements can turn Joe Average into a genius, if he's already eating a balanced diet – don't be taken in by the marketing hype! But how many of us have a diet that's 'perfect'? If your diet is lacking in the nutrients the brain needs, these sub-clinical deficiencies could be holding you back, and in this case improving your diet could certainly help your brain to function at its best.

Many nutrient deficiencies, particularly in their early stages, manifest themselves in symptoms such as fatigue, listlessness and feeling 'out of sorts', and psychological problems such as depression. This is certainly true in the case of vitamin C deficiency (well before you see the symptoms of full-blown scurvy). And iron-deficiency anaemia can impair concentration, making you feel fuzzy-headed – address the iron deficiency, and you'll feel 'brainier'.

NUTRITION AND DEVELOPMENT

Food's impact on the brain begins even before you're born. A developing baby's every nutritional need has to be met by the mother, so her eating habits are crucial.

Particularly important nutrients for building healthy babies are good-quality protein, folic acid, iron, vitamin A, calcium and zinc. And for the developing brain, healthy unsaturated fats are vital – 60 per cent of the brain's dry weight is composed of these fats. The omega-3 and omega-6 essential fatty acids are the most important. The omega-3 docosahexanoic acid (DHA) in particular, and also the omega-6 arachidonic acid (AA), are critical in the brain's structure, together making up about 20 per cent of the brain. DHA is also needed for the developing eye – it makes up 60 per cent of the photoreceptors that pick up light in the eye and transmit messages to the brain.

One recent study looking at mothers' total intake of fish (oily fish is rich in DHA) during pregnancy found benefits from a high intake, in the children's eventual language development. Another study found benefits for children's attention levels.

After the baby is born, the mother's diet continues to affect her child's brain if she is breast-feeding, as breast milk is particularly rich in those essential fatty acids.

As a child grows, develops and becomes an adult, the 'brain-building' EFA, DHA, becomes less important, and is overshadowed by EPA, the 'brain-maintaining' EFA.

EATING TO BENEFIT YOUR BRAIN

A 'brain diet' isn't rocket science – all will be explained in the following chapters. Here, in a nutshell, is what's involved:

- Remove 'junk food'
- Monitor carbohydrates, particularly sugars (which should be minimised)
- Minimise artificial additives
- Look carefully at your intake of caffeine and alcohol
- Increase your intake of essential fatty acids
- Add good, home-cooked foods

- Eat regular meals (breakfast is particularly important)
- Add supplements where necessary
- Some people are allergic or intolerant to certain foods; therefore a test may be required (or for one month avoid products you suspect)

In this chapter we'll quickly run through the nutrients the brain needs for different functions – fuel, brain-building, transmitting messages and the like. Then, in Chapter 11, we'll go into more detail on 'brain foods' and how to incorporate them into your diet. Finally, Chapter 15 will contain a 'brain friendly' eating plan to get you started.

NUTRITION AND BRAIN FUNCTION

To function at its best, the brain needs the right energy supply (glucose) in sufficient quantity. Then, because the brain is constantly being remodelled, and forming new connections between brain cells, it needs the raw materials for this. The brain also needs the components to produce the chemical messengers (neurotransmitters) that send electrical messages around the nervous system. Finally, it needs vitamins and minerals, necessary to make enzymes, and to catalyse (kick-start) many of the metabolic processes within the brain cells.

The brain's energy supply

The brain is an extremely energy-hungry organ – the hungriest in the body. Although it makes up only 2 per cent of an adult's body weight, it demands approximately 20 per cent of their energy supply.

Ultimately, the body's main fuel source is the single-unit sugar, glucose, and the brain relies almost exclusively on this substance for energy. However, the brain (and the rest of the body) likes its energy in a steady stream, not in fits and starts, and one of the keys to ensuring that your brain functions at its full potential is to maintain stable blood-sugar levels.

The digestive system can break down starchy carbohydrates – like bread, pasta and rice – to produce simple sugars. And your liver can synthesise them from other dietary components. The problems occur when you feed your body on neat sugar. When we eat sugar or sugary foods, it's absorbed very quickly, and needs hardly any processing before it can be used as fuel. Our blood-sugar level rises sharply, but all too quickly the fuel is used up, or removed from the bloodstream and stored. This produces an immediate spike in blood sugar (with an accompanying buzz of energy), but soon it plunges again, leaving you hungry, and often tired, irritable and fuzzy-headed too.

When you eat protein, fat or complex carbohydrates (the carbohydrates you find in starchy foods such as bread, rice and pasta, especially the wholegrain kind), the resulting peak in blood sugar is less steep. These foods take longer to be digested, absorbed and metabolised by the body, so the 'fuel' arrives slowly, over a longer time. Rather than getting a quick burst of energy, you feel sustained for longer.

This principle underlies the glycaemic index (GI) concept, which is a key to maximising your brain's potential.

Entire books have been published on the GI principle, but you really only need to remember a few basic concepts.

- The foods that are best for your brain (and also the rest of your body) are the low-GI ones. Remember 'low is slow' – and slow-release foods are what you want.
- Anything that slows the digestion and absorption of a food will lower its GI. Protein is a good example of this. Fat also lowers a meal's GI, but because of the health problems associated with saturated and trans fats, or a high total fat intake, you shouldn't use this as an excuse to overindulge in fatty foods.
- Go for high-fibre foods where possible – fibre lowers the GI. Always choose 'brown' or 'wholemeal' versions, rather than white.
- Processing and cooking raises a food's GI. In effect, you've taken away some of the 'work' the body would have needed to do in order to digest the food, so it can be absorbed faster. Cook vegetables lightly (steaming is best) and don't boil pasta and rice to death. Your food will retain more nutrients too.
- If you eat a low-GI food plus a high-GI food, that makes a medium-GI meal. It's the overall GI of a meal that's important, not the individual foods.

WHAT ABOUT GL?

You might have heard of GL – this stands for glycaemic load, and it's an updated version of GI. One problem with GI is that it gives a high (bad) GI value to some otherwise healthy foods, which puts people off. Sweet-tasting veg, like carrots, are high GI, because of their natural sugars – but you'd have to eat a field's worth to get a blood-sugar spike from carrots!

Glycaemic load considers the *amount* of sugars a serving of food contains. Carrots don't contain much sugar per carrot (thanks to their high water content), so they have a low (good) GL. However, white pasta is very high in starch, which the body rapidly digests to sugar, and it's denser, so white pasta has a higher (worse) GL.

How the Body Controls Blood Sugar

After a meal, food is digested and absorbed, and the level of glucose in the blood rises. This glucose can then be carried in the bloodstream to all of the cells in the body. When the body detects that blood sugar is rising too high, it causes the pancreas to produce the hormone insulin, which squirrels glucose away in cells for use or storage, bringing the blood-sugar level back down. Unchecked, blood glucose could rise to dangerous levels, and this is what happens in untreated diabetes.

The insulin response means that blood glucose cannot rise dangerously high, but even in a healthy person it still allows blood sugar to rise and fall throughout the day. However, the brain functions best when it has a steady, drip-feed of glucose, not a roller coaster of highs and lows, which can lead to various nasty symptoms such as fluctuating energy levels and mood swings. It's the drip-feed effect that we're talking about when we say we want to maintain 'steady blood-sugar levels', and different foods, and combinations of foods, have different effects on blood-sugar levels.

A person's health also affects blood-sugar levels – most notably in the case of untreated diabetes, where the person is unable to control their blood sugar, which rises dangerously high after eating.

However, there is also a condition called impaired glucose tolerance (sometimes called 'pre-diabetes') in which the body's glucose-regulation mechanisms are functioning poorly, allowing blood glucose to rise too high – but not as high as in diabetes.

- When your blood sugar rises higher, you can feel anxious and 'hyper'
- When it is low, you can feel hungry and irritable
- When it is stable, people generally feel calmer

Unstable blood sugar and the brain

Although it doesn't actively do 'work' in the way that muscles do, the brain requires a remarkable amount of energy. Because brain cells (neurons) can't store energy, they need a constant supply, and if your blood-sugar levels fall, the brain gets hungry! Fortunately, the brain is able to look after itself by mobilising energy stores from elsewhere in the body.

Although the brain can keep itself from starving, and maintain the flow of glucose into its cells within set limits, problems can still occur as blood glucose in the brain rises and falls. In other words, even within 'normal' limits, glucose levels that are constantly high, that fall low, or constantly roller-coaster, are not a good idea. If this happens you're likely to experience 'hungry brain' symptoms such as feeling weak, anxious and unable to concentrate.

Links have been found between high sugar intake, unstable blood sugar and behavioural symptoms such as an inability to concentrate and hyperactive or even aggressive behaviour. Eating too much sugar isn't a good idea for anyone – sugar provides 'empty' calories, contributes towards tooth decay, and can increase blood fats. And while a high-sugar diet is problematic for anyone, it's a particularly bad idea for anyone suffering from behaviour or learning difficulties.

Impaired control of blood sugar (though not as serious as that seen in diabetes) is commonly seen in children with ADHD – a study of 265 hyperactive children found that over 75 per cent of them were abnormally poor at maintaining stable blood-sugar levels.

HIGH BLOOD SUGAR AND THE BRAIN

Too much sugar is bad for the brain. A thought-provoking study from New York University Medical Center and School of Medicine suggests that people whose ability to regulate their blood sugar is poor suffer from impaired recent memory, and the area of the brain concerned with memory and learning (the hippocampus) was found to shrink. The research looked at middle-aged and elderly people who did not suffer from diabetes, but had 'impaired glucose tolerance' – pre-diabetes – where blood-sugar regulation is less efficient and blood-sugar levels higher. The scientists suggested that when the brain's energy demands are particularly high (such as while trying to remember something) the glucose levels drop in the parts of the brain doing the work in individuals with impaired glucose tolerance, causing the poor performance in memory tests found by the research.

Studies on diabetics (whose blood-sugar levels rise dangerously high unless controlled by medication, diet and exercise, or a combination) have also shown that too-high blood sugar causes small but significant impairment in cognition (thinking ability). However, the 'hypos' sometimes suffered by diabetics (where the blood sugar falls dangerously low) appear not to cause any long-term harm to the brain.

Amino acids – nutrients for neurotransmitters

As well as needing the proper fuel in the correct amounts, the brain needs protein building blocks (amino acids) in order to make the signalling molecules called neurotransmitters.

The importance of fats

Fats have had a lot of bad press, nutrition-wise, and not without reason. Fat is packed with calories, and too much can cause you to put on weight. Some kinds of fat – the saturated and trans varieties – increase your risk of diseases such as heart disease and cancer. But it's wrong to be fat phobic – there are 'good' fats, and moderate amounts of these are very important for our health.

As stated earlier, the brain is approximately 60 per cent fat. But this isn't any old fat – most of it is the highly unsaturated kind, notably the omega-3 and omega-6 essential fatty acids.

Most of this brain fat is incorporated into cell membranes. Brain-cell membranes need to be flexible in order to function properly, enabling cells to release their neurotransmitters, and then for the receptors to take up these chemical messengers, so that signals can pass between cells. Flexible membranes require fluid fats in their structure, and this means the polyunsaturated omega-3 and omega-6 essential fatty acids, and if the essential fat called DHA is deficient, cell-to-cell signalling can be significantly slowed.

In addition, fats (and also proteins) are needed to manufacture myelin sheaths – a kind of fatty insulating covering for nerve cells. Without this insulation, messages from adjacent nerve cells would cause 'short-circuiting' in the nervous system.

And finally, essential fatty acids are needed to produce hormone-like eicosanoids, which have a wide range of body and brain functions.

The essential fatty acids in the brain are constantly being recycled and replenished, which is why you need to keep topping up your intake of these healthy fats.

Vitamins and minerals for the brain

Vitamins and minerals are known as micronutrients, because we only need them in minute quantities. But they're crucial for our body's healthy functioning – and the brain is no exception.

Our brains need a healthy balanced diet that provides all our daily requirements for vitamins and minerals, to kick-start various chemical reactions, as well as protecting our cells from damage.

Some micronutrients are more important for the brain than others.

B vitamins

The vitamins of the B complex (vitamin B1 or thiamine, vitamin B2 or riboflavin, vitamin B3 or niacin, pyridoxine, vitamin B12, folic acid and biotin) are important in keeping the brain and nervous system healthy. They are also essential during pregnancy, as they are needed for the development of the baby's brain and nervous system.

Iron

We need iron to produce haemoglobin – a pigment found in red blood cells that transports oxygen around the body. Every cell in our body requires oxygen to survive, but the brain is particularly vulnerable to being short of oxygen.

Because of this, if you are deficient in iron your oxygen-transporting capacity will be below par, which can lead to symptoms such as tiredness, lethargy and an inability to concentrate, and have a negative effect on brain function.

Antioxidants

Antioxidants are vitamins, minerals and other compounds found in food that protect the body's cells – including brain cells – from damage by reactive molecules called free radicals. The essential fatty acids in cell membranes are particularly vulnerable to damage from free radicals, so it's vital that they are protected by antioxidants.

Antioxidants also have an important role in keeping our circulatory system healthy, and stopping our blood vessels from becoming clogged or damaged. Blood flow in the brain is crucial, as it is this which enables oxygen and fuel (in the form of glucose) to reach every brain cell.

Examples of antioxidants are vitamins A, C and E, as well as phytochemicals (plant chemicals), which give coloured fruit and vegetables their various hues, plus the polyphenols found in tea and red wine.

Zinc

The mineral zinc is needed for the proper functioning of the brain. It's thought to be particularly important for a region of the brain called the hippocampus, which is involved in memory and learning.

Low levels of zinc have been associated with ADHD in children, and zinc supplements can be effective in treating its symptoms.

Overweight bodies – struggling brains

In terms of brain function, obesity can present a real problem. Being overweight increases your risk of impaired glucose tolerance and poor blood-sugar control, and this makes it all the more important to maintain a healthy weight.

Also, when the results of a recent five-year study on the relationship between body weight and brain function were published, the outcome was worrying, to say the least. The research took two groups of people and gave them tests to measure brain function (psychometric tests) over a five-year period. Group 1 were individuals with a body weight (for their height) in the normal range, while Group 2 was in the range considered obese.

Over the five-year period Group 1 did really well with the brain-function tests while Group 2 showed trends in decline of brain function to such a degree that the press called these results 'The Homer Simpson Effect'.

Meal Patterns

Meal patterns also have an important effect on the way your brain works. Most people are familiar with the feeling that their brain isn't functioning at its best if they skip meals – they feel dizzy or light-headed. Also, if you let yourself get too hungry, you're more likely to crave unhealthy sugary snacks. Regular, moderate-sized meals and healthy snacks keep your energy levels topped up.

Most people report feeling 'slow' and woolly-headed after a big meal, particularly if it's high in starchy carbohydrates. In fact, this 'post-prandial dip' is a well-studied and documented phenomenon. Carbohydrate is probably the main culprit, and adding good-quality (low-fat) protein to a meal lessens this effect, and may even have a slight 'mentally arousing' effect. However, a high fat content in a meal can also lead to a decrease in alertness two to three hours after a meal.

The post-meal dip affects people differently. Your personality matters – anxious people, producing more of the stress hormone, cortisol, suffer less, and the effect is lessened in anyone if they are in a noisy or stimulating environment, or if they have a cup of coffee!

The benefits of breakfast

In terms of blood-sugar maintenance, breakfast is probably the most important meal of the day. When you wake up in the morning, you have gone without food for many hours and your blood sugar will be at its lowest ebb. Skipping breakfast can lower your blood glucose even further, leading to poor concentration, headaches, tiredness and dizziness.

Going without breakfast and grabbing a quick coffee and a dough-nut is no good to man or beast. Breakfast should contain a mix of foods, not just breakfast cereals – it's no good taking on board a processed food that will be digested far too quickly. Instead of that chocolate-coated bar, why not have an apple mid-morning and then opt for a healthy salad at lunchtime? Mid-afternoon another piece of fruit should see you through until it is time for dinner, which should be taken at a time that does not leave you feeling peckish before bedtime.

The effect of whether you have or skip breakfast, and the type of food you eat, has been extensively studied – mostly in children, but also in college students and adults. The results are not always clear cut, but the general consensus is that skipping breakfast interferes with thinking processes, and the ability to learn.

Here are just a few of the benefits of a healthy (low GI, moderate protein) breakfast, drawn from the studies:

- Your blood-sugar level will be more stable during the morning.
- Children eating healthy breakfasts have been found to be less irritable and troublesome in class. Studies on adults are fewer and less conclusive, but many adults report getting annoyed or upset more easily if they skip breakfast, or grab an unhealthy high-GI breakfast that's high in simple sugars.
- Eating a healthy breakfast makes it easier to concentrate and stay alert. Some studies also suggest that an overly large breakfast can decrease the ability to concentrate. However, it did increase memory in some research.
- In studies, children who ate a healthy breakfast scored higher than those who'd skipped breakfast, in a test given late morning.
- Giving children a healthy breakfast sustains them through the morning, so they're less likely to want unhealthy snacks at morning break time. The same is likely to hold true for adults.
- Breakfast eaters are also less likely to overeat during the rest of the day.
- Breakfast can help children maintain a healthy weight. Studies have shown that breakfast skippers are more likely to put on pounds.

In addition, a healthy breakfast provides energy for physical activity, and makes it easier for you to meet your nutrient requirements for the day. Missing breakfast makes it much harder to make up the 'lost' nutrients later in the day.

Slimming diets

Slimming diets that greatly restrict food choice and calorie intake have been shown to hamper mental performance. Crash diets are a bad idea nutritionally speaking – they can lead to nutrient deficiencies, fail to supply sufficient energy, and leave the immune system vulnerable. But not only that – they also stop your brain from functioning at its best.

FOOD FOR THE BRAIN

Good nutrition is important for energy, growth and repair of the body's cells, as well as reducing your risk of illness. And, as we've already mentioned, food plays an important role in the development and function of the brain. But while good nutrition is crucial for everyone, it's even more important for people with any kind of learning or behavioural difficulty.

You can fail to fulfil your full mental potential simply because you are deficient in certain nutrients, or eating too much of certain foods. A diet full of junk food, unhealthy fats, sugar and salt will starve your brain of the raw materials it needs, and 'poison' it with harmful artificial additives and 'anti-nutrients'. Once you know the foods to eat, and which to avoid, you can maximise your brain's potential, not to mention helping you to stay healthy, full of energy, and lose weight if you need to. You simply need to emphasise slow-release wholegrain carbohydrates, quality protein, healthy fats, fruit and vegetables and plenty of water.

BRAIN FATS

You're probably well aware that fats – some kinds at least – can be bad for us, piling on the pounds, and increasing our risk of heart disease, diabetes and cancer. These 'bad' fats are the saturated and hydrogenated fats we'll cover in more detail later.

But our bodies (and brains) need moderate amounts of 'good' fats, and these fats are described as 'unsaturated'. The secret is to make sure that we don't eat too much fat in total, and that the fat we do eat is the healthy unsaturated kind.

As a rule, unsaturated fats are oils – they're liquid at room temperature.

They can be divided into:

- Monounsaturated fats
- Polyunsaturated fats

Monounsaturated fats (monounsaturates)

These include olive oil, canola oil, peanut oil, sesame oil and avocado oil.

Polyunsaturated fats (polyunsaturates)

These include sunflower oil, safflower oil, corn oil and fish oils.

The most important polyunsaturated fats are the omega-3 and omega-6 essential fatty acids (EFAs) – they're called essential because our bodies can't make them, so we have to get them from our diet.

Children with learning and behaviour disorders are generally found to be deficient in omega-3 and omega-6 EFAs, and a lot of research has been done in this area, with encouraging results when the children's intake was supplemented.

Most people don't get enough omegas, but this lack is particularly notable in children and adults with developmental delay syndromes.

If you have any of the following symptoms, you could be lacking in 'brain fats'.

Physical symptoms:

- Dry skin, especially if it looks 'pimply' or rough
- Dry hair
- Dandruff
- Soft or brittle nails
- Itchy, dry eyes
- Raised blood pressure
- Raised cholesterol

'Brain-related' symptoms:

- Learning and behaviour difficulties
- Poor concentration
- Poor short-term memory
- Clumsiness

Omega-3 essential fatty acids

These fats are fantastic for your heart and blood vessels, helping to control your cholesterol levels and reduce your risk of life-threatening blood clots. And when it comes to brain fats, omega-3s really shine. As well as being essential for building brain cells, they're also needed for the day-to-day functioning of the brain. They can also help prevent and fight depression, and help prevent dementia. Unfortunately, many of us don't eat enough of them, especially the highly unsaturated fatty acids EPA and DHA.

The best sources of omega-3s (and especially EPA and DHA) are oily fish, such as salmon, mackerel, pilchards, sardines and fresh tuna (the tuna canning process removes most of the omega-3s). Vegetarians can get lesser amounts from flaxseeds (linseeds) or flaxseed oil, or vegetarian omega-3 supplements.

Omega-6 essential fatty acids:

These beneficial oils have similar, though slightly lesser, heart health effects to omega-3s, and could also reduce our risk of type-2 diabetes, and improve skin conditions such as eczema.

You'll find them in nuts and seeds, as well as corn oil, sunflower oil and safflower oil.

THE FAT BALANCE

Today in the UK, most of us eat too much of the unhealthy saturated fats, and not enough of the healthy polyunsaturated fats the brain needs. In addition to crowding out the good fats from our diets, bad (saturated and trans) fats also directly stop the brain making proper use of the good fats.

Protein

Getting enough protein is rarely a problem in the UK – the issue is the quality. Unfortunately, many of us rely heavily on 'processed protein' – manufactured foods such as sausages, burgers and high-fat ready-meals that are high in unhealthy saturated fat, salt and additives. Also, a lot of people eat more red meat than they should. Red meat is higher in saturated fat than other meats, and it's also linked with a higher risk of certain cancers.

It's fine to eat red meat once or twice a week, but you should aim to concentrate instead on poultry, fish, eggs, and low-fat dairy products such as skimmed milk, yoghurt, cottage cheese and quark. Vegetarian protein sources include pulses (beans and lentils), nuts and seeds, Quorn, and soya products such as tofu and soya meat substitutes.

There are advantages and disadvantages to both animal and non-animal protein sources. Animal protein is a concentrated protein source, which is easiest for the body to use, but it's higher in saturated fat. Vegetarian protein is harder for the body to use, but it lacks the bad saturated fat, and also contain healthy unsaturated fats. They also contain fibre, which is good for digestion, and reduces your heart-disease risk too.

It's probably healthiest to get our protein from as wide a variety of sources as possible and, because the UK diet is rather meat-orientated, this means increasing the vegetable protein for most of us.

> Protein has the added benefit of lowering the glycaemic index of a meal, reducing the 'spike' it causes in your blood-sugar level and sustaining you for longer.

Vitamins and Minerals

As well as protein, carbohydrates and 'good fats', our bodies and brains also need vitamins and minerals. We've already introduced the key players where brain function is concerned (see Chapter 10), but for optimum health (including brain health) you need the whole range of micronutrients. In fact, the first signs of many nutrient deficiencies (including vitamins B2, B12 and C) are low mood and irritability.

Most people can get all the vitamins and minerals they need from a balanced diet, but people suffering from various illnesses, and also from learning difficulties, may have lower levels, or higher requirements. In these cases, supplements may be necessary, and we'll discuss this later in this book.

But it would be wrong to rely on supplements for your micronutrients – they should be 'supplements', not a substitute for a healthy diet. Try to get most of your vitamins and minerals from real food.

Vitamins

Vitamin A (for healthy skin, and vision): get it from meat (especially liver), oily fish, dairy products, eggs, and green, yellow and orange fruit and vegetables.

Vitamin D (for healthy bones and teeth): get it from oily fish (e.g. salmon, sardines, mackerel), meat, eggs and dairy products. A chemical reaction in our bodies also makes vitamin D by the action of sunlight on the skin – about fifteen minutes a day during the summer is enough for most people. Vitamin D is also added to margarines and low-fat spreads, and fortified breakfast cereals.

Vitamin E (for healthy reproductive and immune systems): get it from nuts and seeds, wholegrains, wheatgerm, avocado, spinach and broccoli.

Vitamin K (to enable our blood to clot, and for healthy bones): get it from eggs, fish oils, dairy products and green leafy vegetables.

Vitamins B1, B2 and B3 (also known as thiamin, riboflavin and niacin) have many functions, including helping to release energy from food: get them from meat, wholegrains, nuts, seeds and dark-green leafy vegetables.

Vitamin B6 (for releasing energy from food; it may also help to regulate our moods): get it from meat, beans, potatoes, wholegrains, wheatgerm, nuts and dark-green leafy vegetables.

Folic acid (also known as folate, this B vitamin supports the immune system, helps prevent neural-tube defects in the baby during pregnancy, and helps prevent a kind of anaemia): get it from liver, eggs, green leafy vegetables, pulses and nuts.

Vitamin B12 (for the production of red blood cells): get it from red meat, fish, shellfish, eggs and dairy products (not found in vegan foods, but produced in small amounts by harmless bacteria in our guts).

Vitamin C (for a strong immune system, and wound healing; it also boosts the body's absorption of iron from food): get it from fruit (especially kiwi fruit, blackcurrants, strawberries, citrus fruits), yellow and red peppers, and tomatoes.

Minerals

Iron (for making healthy red blood cells and carrying oxygen around the body; a deficiency can lead to anaemia): get it from liver (the best source), kidney, red meat, chicken, eggs, pulses, green vegetables and dried fruit (especially apricots).

Calcium (for healthy bones and teeth): get it from dairy products, tinned fish where the bones are eaten (e.g. sardines and salmon), tofu, sesame seeds and almonds.

Magnesium (to help the body deal with stress, and for healthy muscles and bones): get it from meat, dairy products, green vegetables, nuts, seeds and pulses.

Potassium (for controlling blood pressure): get it from nuts, seeds, bananas, lentils and green leafy vegetables.

Zinc (for a healthy immune system, growth and development, and sperm formation in men; it also appears to be important in brain function): get it from meat, fish, shellfish, chicken, eggs, dairy products, nuts and seeds.

THE RIGHT CARBOHYDRATES

To keep your blood-sugar levels stable and help provide a steady supply of energy for your brain, you need the right kind of carbohydrates, namely low glycaemic index (GI) starchy carbohydrates, especially wholegrains. When it comes to providing steady, slow-release energy, the 'browner' a carbohydrate the better. Refining grains to make them 'white' dramatically speeds up the rate at which they hit your bloodstream, making them almost as detrimental to balanced blood sugar as pure sugar. Refining also strips away much of the goodness in grains, by removing much of their fibre, vitamins, minerals and protein. In many cases, refined grains are more or less pure starch.

Good carbohydrates include:

- wholemeal bread
- wholemeal pasta
- brown rice

You might also like to give more unusual grains a try, such as millet, buckwheat, bulgur wheat and brown couscous.

Potatoes are also starchy carbohydrates, and are especially nutritious if you eat the skins. But don't undo your good nutritional work by deep-frying them – in other words eating them as chips or crisps. It's far better to bake old potatoes in their jackets, split and fill with a low-fat filling, or roughly 'crush' them (the trendy modern take on mashed potatoes!) or cut them into wedges or chunky chips and bake them. Little new potatoes can be boiled in their skins.

SUCH A THING AS 'GOOD' SUGARS?

We know that refined sugar produces an undesirable, rapid and short-lived spike in blood sugar, with no nutritional benefit. But not all sugar-containing foods are bad. The natural sugars in fruit and the lactose (milk sugar) found in milk don't have the same harmful effects as refined sugar. In the case of fruit, for example, the fibre in the skin and flesh slows the sugar's absorption, turning it from a 'fast-release' fuel like the sugar in sweets or fizzy drinks, to the kind of slow-release fuel that the brain thrives on. As an added bonus, the fruit sugars also come packaged with a whole variety of vitamins, minerals and phytochemicals. Low-fat dairy products are a rich source of protein and calcium.

When choosing fruit, try to minimise their effect on your blood sugar by picking those that are less intensely sweet. In general, tropical fruits (such as pineapple, mango and bananas) raise your blood sugar more rapidly than fruits grown in temperate climates (such as apples, pears and cherries).

Dried fruit is high in fibre (like all fruit), but during the drying process the sugar is concentrated, so dried fruits such as raisins produce a speedier rise in blood sugar than their fresh equivalents. Combining dried fruit with a little protein (such as a few nuts), and only eating a little at a time, helps to decrease the concentrated fruit sugar's impact on blood-sugar levels.

FIBRE

Fibre, once known as 'roughage', has a less than glamorous image, but it's vital for health. The insoluble fibre found in wholegrains, vegetables and fruit (especially the skins) can't be digested by the body, so it bulks up the food in your digestive system, giving the intestines something to 'work on', and helps to prevent diarrhoea and constipation. There's also another type of fibre, called soluble fibre; as well as aiding digestion, it can help lower cholesterol levels. It also helps promote a feeling of fullness between meals, and helps prevent blood-sugar levels from rising too rapidly. This makes it particularly important in preventing blood-sugar-related brain symptoms. Good sources of soluble fibre include oats, fruit (especially apples), peas, beans and lentils.

Because fibre is concentrated in plant sources, the best way to incorporate it into your diet is to eat plenty of plant-based foods – wholegrains, fruit, vegetables and nuts. If you're not used to eating a lot of high-fibre foods, go slowly, as suddenly increasing your fibre intake could make you feel uncomfortable and bloated until your digestive system gets used to it.

> A Swedish study showed that eating a low-GI, high-fibre, carbohydrate-rich breakfast kept blood-sugar levels nice and low for up to ten hours. The low-GI breakfast eaters in the study also scored better in tests of short-term memory.

WATER

Since water makes up about 80 per cent of the brain, it stands to reason that keeping hydrated has a big implication for mental function.

Even a small degree of dehydration can make you feel below par and headachey, with significant implications for your mental performance, concentration and memory. In fact, many of the symptoms of dehydration are related to the effect of water deprivation on the brain.

No one should wait until they're thirsty before drinking. By the time you're thirsty, you're on the way to dehydration. Adults need approximately one and a half to two litres of water a day, which is approximately eight to ten tall glasses.

Plain water is the ultimate hydrator, and herbal and fruit teas are good too. Tea and coffee add to your fluid intake, but as they're also diuretics, some of this benefit is cancelled out. Fruit juice also contributes fluid, but it's high in high-GI sugars, so dilute it half-and-half with water. Fruit squashes and fizzy drinks are packed full of sugar and/or artificial sweeteners and other additives, with little or no nutritional value whatsoever.

Look carefully at the contents of all drinks – many contain high sugar levels and/or aspartame (E951) or saccharine (E945).

CAN YOU SPOT THE PROBLEMS WITH THIS DIET?

Have a look at the list of food items below provided by a patient as a typical day's intake of food and guess what you think might be wrong with it:

- Breakfast – cereal and/or toast and jam with two cups of tea with two sugars
- Mid-morning – cup of coffee with two sugars and a chocolate-covered bar
- Lunch – ham sandwich, packet of crisps and a diet cola
- Mid-afternoon – cup of tea with two sugars and two biscuits
- Evening meal – pasta with carbonara sauce and two glasses of wine

Correct – it is laden with carbohydrates, has limited protein and is totally devoid of any fruit or vegetables. If we now highlight the carbohydrates and other sources of sugars the list will look like this:

- Breakfast – **cereal** and/or **toast** and **jam** with two cups of tea with two **sugars**
- Mid-morning – cup of coffee with two **sugars** and a **chocolate-covered bar**
- Lunch – ham **sandwich**, packet of **crisps** and a **diet cola**
- Mid-afternoon – cup of tea with two **sugars** and two **biscuits**
- Evening meal – **pasta** with carbonara sauce and two **glasses of wine**

Although we do need to have carbohydrates in our daily intake of food, this should be just a part of a balanced diet and not the mainstay. Also, hidden within the list above are trans fats, which do need to be limited.

ANTI-NUTRIENTS

In contrast to the healthy wholefoods already described, with their low-fat protein, low-GI carbohydrates, unsaturated fats and abundance of vitamins and minerals, a lot of the typical UK diet is less than helpful to the brain.

'Junk food', and processed food that's high in fat, sugar, salt and unnecessary artificial additives, can negatively affect the brain's functioning. (High quantities of calorific and fatty foods can also lead to obesity, with all its associated health problems). These foods are also low in the 'brain nutrients' we need to perform to our full mental potential.

CONVENIENCE FOODS

Although a lot of convenience foods are over-processed, high in unhealthy ingredients and lacking in nutrients, some supermarket staples are convenient, without sacrificing good nutrition. For example, you can stock up on tinned tomatoes, reduced-sugar reduced-salt baked beans, other tinned beans, frozen fruit and vegetables, good-quality low-fat salad cream and mayonnaise, fruit spreads (rather than jam), and reduced-sugar reduced-salt peanut butter, with a clear conscience.

Before you put anything in your basket or trolley, check its saturated fat, sugar, salt and additive content. Also see whether the ingredients list contains anything you wouldn't expect to see, such as a high water or sugar content in sliced meat.

ADDITIVES

With the advent of white goods, the fridge and freezer have replaced the larder and pantry, and food that would have lasted no more than a day or two can be stored safely for months. With a microwave and a ready-to-eat meal it's no longer seen as necessary to be able to cook, and a meal that could take an hour or more to prepare and cook can be ready in minutes. Not only can you have meals that virtually cook themselves, it is also possible to have pretty well anything you want at any time, day or night. However, all this convenience comes at a price and it is not just paying through the nose for organic produce that increases the cost of our food. In order to have all these ready-made products just waiting for us to choose from, they all need a long shelf life. Also, as we want all these wonderful products to look their best, all fresh and inviting, the vast majority contain one or two things to keep them looking that way – chemicals in the form of artificial additives such as preservatives.

It's impossible to avoid additives totally. Without preservatives, for example, we would be at high risk of serious food poisoning. But it's a good idea for anyone – and especially those with a developmental delay syndrome such as those described in this book – to avoid *unnecessary* chemicals, as several of these have been implicated in brain-related symptoms (and other negative health effects, such as increasing asthma symptoms).

The use of food additives has increased dramatically and they are now found not just in food but also in products such as toothpaste and medications. It is my belief, and that of a great many serious scientists, that there is a very real link between food additives and behavioural problems – especially in the case of ADHD sufferers, but also in other behaviour and learning problems, as well as anxiety, depression, schizophrenia and Alzheimer's disease.

For years individuals and organisations alike have campaigned against the use of certain E numbers in food and drink. A little research will show you that many E numbers that are permitted in the UK are banned in other countries around the world and that until very recently E numbers were only tested in isolation. That is, even though we eat a cocktail of E numbers each day, until very recently no one had thought to check to see if this is safe. Now, of course, we know that this daily cocktail of E numbers could well be damaging our health and may be playing a huge role in the epidemic rise in developmental delay in children.

If you are healthy and have no learning or behavioural problems you should still eat healthily and avoid these bad E numbers, but if you do have any developmental delay issues then I believe it is essential that you take bad E numbers very seriously and as far as possible eliminate them from your diet. The logic is simple – if your brain is struggling to cope on a daily basis with the demands of life, then why add to that stress by eating 8 to 9 pounds (around 4kg) of chemicals that have been shown in combination to have neurotoxic (brain-poisoning) properties?

The main types of additives are:

- Antioxidants
- Colours
- Emulsifiers, stabilisers, gelling agents and thickeners
- Flavourings and flavour enhancers
- Preservatives
- Sweeteners

They are used to make food:

- Look and taste better
- Stay fresh for longer
- More nutritious (for example by adding vitamins, or probiotic friendly bacteria)
- Cheaper to manufacture

Salt is an additive, used to keep food fresh and improve its taste. So is sugar. While both of these should be minimised in our diets, they are not what people generally mean by 'additives'. What we mean are the artificial additives with complex chemical names, and often E numbers.

E numbers in themselves are nothing to be afraid of – they mean that the chemical has been tested and judged to be safe and nontoxic. Some vitamins, such as vitamin C, have been designated E numbers for when they're added to foods.

But other additives are potentially more sinister. Although they have been judged safe in normal doses, there's less evidence about their effects in combination and over long periods of time – which is how, in reality, we eat them.

There's plenty of anecdotal evidence supporting the link between diet and behaviour. Most of this concerns children, as the effect on their smaller, developing bodies is more marked, but adults often also see an improvement in mental symptoms when they 'clean up' their diet and dump the unnecessary additives. This is especially noticeable when the symptoms are related to hyperactive behaviour and/or mood swings.

Flavourings and flavour enhancers

Over 4,500 artificial flavourings are permitted in our foods, but they don't have to be named on the label – all you will see there is 'flavourings'. We don't even need them – they're generally only added to food that doesn't contain much of the 'real' ingredients that would give it taste. For example, a yoghurt that is low in real fruit needs to contain artificial flavourings in order to make it taste fruity.

Far better to avoid flavourings where possible, and eat food that gets its taste from natural ingredients.

Flavour enhancers are added to foods to make the taste they do contain seem stronger. Monosodium glutamate (MSG or E621) is the most familiar. Its active ingredient is glutamic acid, or glutamate, which is naturally found in foods including Parmesan cheese, tomatoes and plums. Glutamic acid is a neurotransmitter, toxic in high doses, but it's usually consumed in sufficiently small quantities for the body to deal with. However, if you eat a lot of additive-containing foods, you may take in too much glutamic acid (naturally from food *plus* added in the form of MSG). MSG isn't a problem for most people, but in some it can cause symptoms including asthma, runny nose, headaches, palpitations and behavioural symptoms such as hyperactivity.

Also, glutamate-containing additives have been implicated in what has been called 'glutamate storms', which are important to people suffering from developmental delay syndromes. These additives seem to trigger a cascade effect, churning out too much of the excitatory neurotransmitter glutamate, and this has been seen to cause hyperactive and often pointless destructive behaviour in children.

Artificial sweeteners

Artificial sweeteners are commonly added to 'diet' and low-calorie foods, as well as 'diabetic' foods, as they have a fraction of the calories, and less impact on blood sugar, than true sugars. They are also cheaper than 'real' sugar, so manufacturers add them to many non-diet foods where sugar would otherwise be used.

Many people are attempting to minimise their intake of artificial sweeteners – although there is no evidence proving they are harmful to humans when eaten in normal quantities, some animal studies have implicated these chemicals in increasing cancer risk, and anecdotal reports have linked them with behavioural changes such as hyperactivity, aggression, anxiety, depression, mood swings and also migraine.

The commonest artificial sweeteners are:

- **Aspartame (E951):** The best-known (and most infamous) artificial sweetener, alleged to contribute to a variety of health problems. Food manufacturers point out that no research has proven a link between aspartame and ill health, but it's probably not worth taking the risk, especially if you suffer from any behaviour or learning problems. Avoid labels bearing the words: aspartame, E951, Nutrasweet™, Equal™, Canderel™, Spoonful™, Benevia™ or 'contains a source of phenylalanine'.

    Probably even more than MSG, aspartame has been implicated in 'glutamate storms', with their resultant hyperactive behaviour.

- **Saccharin (E954):** this is the oldest sugar substitute. Depending upon who you believe (manufacturers or consumer advocates), it is either perfectly safe or a cancer risk.

- **Acesulfame K (E950):** Implicated in brain-related symptoms such as blurred vision.

- **Sucralose (E955, or Splenda™):** Based on current research, this is one of the safer additives.

- **Xylitol (E967):** Seems less risky than other sweeteners – probably the best of a bad bunch.

ASPARTAME – A CHEQUERED HISTORY

A little surfing on the internet will soon bring you to a host of allegations that include aspartame being linked to brain tumours, seizures, birth defects, multiple sclerosis, headaches and dizziness.

A slim chance of the truth

For adults in particular there is also the possibility of unwittingly consuming copious amounts of aspartame as part of a misguided attempt to get fit by losing weight. By choosing to buy products that are sugar-free or contain no added sugar as part of your calorie-controlled diet, you are probably ingesting vast quantities of aspartame. If you really want to be health-conscious you might want to think about taking a magnifying glass with you the next time you visit the supermarket and look out for E951 – the E number for aspartame. While doing this, ask yourself a simple question: why would a manufacturer go to the bother and expense of changing the details on the packaging? Could it be that they are a little concerned about using the word 'aspartame' and, if so, I wonder why?

Colourings

The strongest link between additives and brain and behavioural symptoms is for artificial colourings (along with the preservative sodium benzoate). A lot of high-quality research has been conducted on children's behaviour when artificial colourings are removed from their diets. Most recently, the Food Standards Agency commissioned research at Southampton University, where two groups of children (aged three and nine) were given drinks containing two different cocktails of colourings plus the preservative sodium benzoate, or natural fruit juice. All of the drinks looked and tasted identical, and neither the children and their parents, nor the people giving out the drinks, knew which was which.

The researchers then studied the children's behaviour, based on reports from teachers and parents and, for the older children, a computer-based test of attention.

When the results were analysed, both of the colourings mixes were found to increase hyperactive behaviour, compared with the pure fruit drink. Interestingly, unlike many other similar studies, the children tested were taken from a cross-section of the population, and not all of them suffered from attention deficit problems such as ADHD. However, the effects were stronger in the children diagnosed with hyperactivity disorders.

In the wake of this important study, the Food Standards Agency (FSA) has advised parents whose children show signs of hyperactivity that they might see improvement if they remove the additives used in the study from their children's diets.

The colourings used were:

● Sunset yellow (E110)
● Quinoline yellow (E104)

- Carmoisine (E122)
- Allura red (E129)
- Tartrazine (E102)
- Ponceau 4R (E124)

Also used was the preservative sodium benzoate (E211).

And since the evidence against these colours is so strong, cutting them out would seem very good advice for anyone with learning or behavioural difficulties, or indeed any member of the population.

Preservatives

Humans have used food preservatives for thousands of years, adding salt (as in salt fish and bacon) and sugar (as in jams) to food to enable it to be stored. But, although we should decrease the salt and sugar in our diets, when we talk about preservatives, we generally mean the artificial chemicals added by the food industry.

Sodium benzoate (E211) is probably the priority to avoid. One of the chemicals in the Southampton hyperactivity study, it is also implicated in conditions including asthma. When combined with vitamin C (also labelled as ascorbic acid or E300), for example in many soft drinks, it can produce benzene, which can trigger cancer.

Other common food preservatives include sulphur dioxide (E220) and other sulphites, which are implicated in worsening asthma, and possibly heart and lung conditions. They are used in manufactured fruit products and drinks, and also sausage meat.

THE DIRTY DOZEN CHEMICALS

The organic baby-food company Organix produced a *Carrots or Chemistry* report that came up with a 'Dirty Dozen' additives parents should avoid in their children's food – unsurprisingly, it included most of the colourings in the Southampton study. We believe that for anyone who is trying to minimise the potentially harmful chemicals they take in with their food, these two lists are a good place to start.

1. Monosodium glutamate (flavouring) E621
2. Sodium 5-ribonucleotide (flavouring) E625

3.   Aspartame (sweetener) E951
4.   Acesulphame K (sweetener) E950
5.   Sodium saccharine (sweetener) E954
6.   Sodium benzoate (preservative) E220
7.   Quinoline yellow (colouring) E104
8.   Brilliant blue (colouring) E133
9.   Sunset yellow (colouring) E110
10. Carmoisine (colouring) E122
11. Ponceau 4R (colouring) E124
12. Indigo carmine (colouring) E132

Campaigners at the Food Commission have set up a very useful website with a database of products containing suspect ingredients: www.actiononadditives.com

What Can Be Done?

More and more research is telling us that some food additives are very bad news. But has the government called for urgent action, are backbenchers up in arms? I think not.

However, on a more encouraging note, a report by the Associate Parliamentary Food and Health Forum has made several recommendations including:

● Commissioning more research on nutrition and the brain, especially determining the optimum intakes of omega-3 essential fatty acids at different stages of life
● More trials of nutritional supplements in Young Offender Institutes
● Nutritional standards for prison meals (similar to those seen already for school meals)
● Banning artificial colourings, and nonessential preservatives, from foods and soft drinks

But of the people who could make a huge difference to what we eat and more importantly what is in what we eat, the manufacturers are the least likely to act. They are in business to make a profit and would quite rightly say that they are feeding a demand. That they are potentially feeding an educational and social crisis is perhaps too much for them to own up to.

Retailers, particularly the supermarket giants, could force the manufacturers to come into line, but it would take a very brave board of directors to take such an ethical stance. However, if one supermarket were to take that giant step for mankind, the others would be forced to follow. Parliament could bring about such a change, but who would have the foresight to see not only the health benefits such a change could bring about but also the huge financial savings that could be made in terms of education, disability allowance, policing, the courts, the prison service, hospitals, etc., not to mention putting an end to so much suffering.

You and Me

One lady I came across had a very novel idea and that was simply to return products to the supermarket that contained artificial sweeteners and/or additives and say to the manager that the product made her feel unwell. If enough people did this, the supermarket might get the message very quickly and that message would very soon reach the ears of the manufacturers.

If we are going to make a change, it is going to have to be you and me that make it happen, for we have a vested interest in our health and that of our children, while the manufacturers might well have other agendas.

SUGAR

In the UK we eat more sugar than we should – the average intake for men is around 40 per cent too high, and 21 per cent too much for women. And the sweetest-toothed people eat far more than those average figures.

Everyone should cut down their refined sugar intake – and especially those with developmental delay conditions.

Daily Sugar Intakes in the UK

	Actual (average)	Recommended maximum
Men	87g	64g
Women	57g	47g

In order to cut down, you need to know your enemy. Some sugary foods are obvious, such as sweets, chocolates, fizzy drinks, biscuits, cakes, ice cream and other desserts. But you'll also find sugar 'hidden' in many foods that don't taste sweet, such as table sauces, chutneys and pickles, non-sweetened breakfast cereals (e.g. cornflakes and bran flakes) and even processed meat products (where sugar can be used to 'hold' water in the meat, in order to bulk it out).

If you want to avoid hidden sugar, you'll need to read the food labels.

Anything containing more than 10g sugars per 100g is considered a high-sugar food by the Food Standards Agency. Look instead for foods with what they'd say is 'a little' sugar – in other words 2g of sugar or less per 100g.

Nutrition claims on packaging also provides clues on a food's sugar content – though they can be misleading. For example, 'reduced sugar' means 30 per cent less sugar than the 'standard' version – though it could still be a high-sugar food. 'Low sugar' means no more than 5g sugars per 100g for foods (and no more than 2.5g sugars per 100ml for drinks), and 'sugar-free' products are allowed no more than 0.5g sugars per 100g or 100ml.

You'll also need to know the many names used for sugars – you'll notice that many end in '-ose'. The higher they appear on the ingredients list, the more of them you'll find in the food.

- Sucrose
- Fructose
- Glucose
- Fructose
- Lactose
- Maltose
- Dextrose
- Treacle
- Honey
- Golden syrup
- Corn syrup
- Maple syrup
- Invert sugar
- Raw sugar
- Hydrolysed starch

You can also reduce your sugar intake by swapping high-sugar foods for lower-sugar alternatives – try these sugar swaps:

High-sugar snacks: Biscuits, cakes, chocolate, sweets
Lower-sugar alternatives: Malt loaf, currant buns, wholemeal scones, plain popcorn, fruit, nuts, seeds

High-sugar breakfasts: Sugary breakfast cereals (including corn-flakes and bran flakes), Danish pastries
Lower-sugar alternatives: Porridge with mashed banana or a teaspoon of honey to sweeten, beans on toast, scrambled or poached egg on toast.

High-sugar desserts: Ready-prepared desserts and puddings, ice cream, bought fruit yoghurts, canned fruit in syrup
Lower-sugar alternatives: Home-made low-sugar desserts such as baked apple, summer pudding, yoghurt with fruit, pancakes with fresh fruit and yoghurt, canned fruit in juice, or fresh or frozen fruit

High-sugar drinks: Sugary fizzy drinks, milkshakes, squash, regular hot chocolate
Lower-sugar alternatives: Water, pure juice diluted with water or sparkling water, tea, diluted fruit juice, home-made smoothies using yoghurt and fresh fruit, hot chocolate using milk and a very small quantity of good-quality drinking chocolate

Other high-sugar foods: 'Regular' tomato ketchup, canned sweet corn, baked beans and spaghetti
Lower-sugar alternatives: Low-sugar ketchup, low-sugar canned sweet corn, baked beans and spaghetti

---

PURE JUICE

Pure fruit juice is full of vitamins, but it's also high in sugar, in a quick-release form that rapidly hits your bloodstream. It's far better to get your fruity vitamins from eating the whole fruit, and when you want a fruity drink, dilute pure juice half-and-half with water.

Eventually, try to wean yourself off sweet tastes – it *is* possible, just take it slowly. Gradually cut down the sugar you take in drinks, have diluted fruit juice rather than sugar-laden fizz, and swap your sugary snacks for higher-fibre alternatives with less of a sweet taste. In a few months' time, you'll find that your old 'treats' taste sickly sweet.

Don't rely on artificial sweeteners to reduce your sugar load. On top of the possible bad reactions to these chemicals seen in some people with developmental delay disorders, they do nothing to blunt your sweet tooth – which is what we ultimately want to achieve.

BAD FATS

Unsaturated fats are good for us, and omega-3s and -6s are absolutely vital. But saturated, hydrogenated and trans fats have nothing to recommend them.

Saturated fats are the kind found in animal products, such as meat, dairy products and eggs. They're also found in certain tropical oils, such as palm oil (palm fat). These are the kind of fats that contribute to raised cholesterol levels, clogged arteries, raised blood pressure, and an increased risk of heart disease, strokes and cancer.

As well as these health risks, saturated fats also have implications for brain function, because of the artery-clogging effects. Because the brain is such a 'hungry' organ, it needs a huge blood supply, and if the arteries and capillaries supplying it aren't smooth, clear and stretchy, the brain suffers. In the worst-case scenario, a blood vessel is blocked or ruptures, resulting in a stroke. But anything that hinders blood flow is bad for the brain.

We need to remember, though, that although animal products are the main source of saturated fat, meat, dairy products and eggs are still rich sources of important nutrients such as protein, fat-soluble vitamins including A and E, and several important minerals such as iron, calcium and zinc. You don't have to give up animal products, but it is a good idea to minimise your fat intake from them by:

- Choosing the least fatty cuts of meat, and removing visible fat
- Avoiding fast food and processed food, which often relies on cheaper, fattier meat
- Removing the skin from poultry – this is where you find most of the fat

- Buying low-fat dairy products, such as skimmed or semi-skimmed milk, low-fat natural yoghurt, low-fat cream cheese and cottage cheese
- Going easy on the full-fat cheese – if you use smaller quantities of stronger cheeses, such as Parmesan, you can use less, and cut the saturated fat

If saturated fats are bad, hydrogenated fats are even worse. Hydrogenated fats are the main source of trans fats in our diets. Trans fats have the same dreadful effects on the heart and blood vessels as saturated fats, and are also believed to crowd out the crucial omegas in their role in brain structure and function.

Hydrogenated fats (or hydrogenated oils) are an invention of the food industry, who take otherwise healthy oils and harden them to make produce cheap fats with a long shelf life. These go into a wide variety of products, including ready-meals, sauces in packets and jars, 'instant' mixes such as soups, drinks and desserts, bought cakes and cake mixes, biscuits, pastries, sweets, desserts, some ice creams, chocolates and chocolate bars. They are sometimes used for frying in fast-food outlets.

Fortunately, the food industry has responded to public pressure to remove these 'Frankenfats' from our food, and many companies and supermarkets are phasing them out of their products. This makes it even more important to read the labels and avoid those that are dragging their feet about removing the harmful fats, and look out for 'trans fat free' flashes on the packaging.

And ultimately, the best way to minimise the trans fats in your diet is to keep it simple, and to make as much as possible from scratch.

> You won't see 'trans fats' on the labels – look for the word 'hydrogenated' or 'partially hydrogenated' vegetable fats or oils instead. This means that a food will have trans fats in it.

Stimulant Foods and Drinks

Stimulants, including those found in food and drinks, unbalance blood sugar. The caffeine in coffee, cola and chocolate trigger a release of the hormone adrenaline, which primes the body for action, causing the release of more glucose into the bloodstream.

Chocolate provides a double-whammy to blood-sugar levels – not only is it high in sugar, it also contains caffeine, plus a weaker stimulant called theobromine.

When you habitually eat or drink stimulants, your body becomes accustomed to them, so that you need to keep consuming them just to feel 'normal', creating a vicious cycle. You may even find you need more to gain the same 'buzz' – this is particularly noted in coffee drinkers.

Try to reduce the amount of stimulants in your diet, especially if you suffer from developmental delay symptoms.

Sources of caffeine:

- Cup of brewed coffee   90mg caffeine
- Cup of instant coffee   60mg caffeine
- Cup of tea   40mg caffeine
- Can of cola   up to 70mg caffeine
- Can of energy drink   up to 70mg caffeine
- 50g chocolate bar   10mg caffeine.
- Cup of hot chocolate   5mg caffeine

Many painkillers and cold cures also contain caffeine, so check the labels.

ALCOHOL

Alcohol may make you feel confident and outgoing, but it's actually a depressant. There's a very fine line between that 'happy' feeling and slowed reactions and sleepiness. And if you drink too much, too often, you can do long-term harm to your body.

The recommended maximum amount of alcohol for men is 21 units per week, or 14 for women, with at least two alcohol-free days per week. And you mustn't save up all your units for a marathon weekend drinking session, as this is what counts as binge drinking!

However, moderate drinking is associated with better health than being teetotal, and that moderate amount seems to be about half to one glass per day.

A 2007 study in the *British Medical Journal* last year showed that men aged 50 to 65 who had a drink every day had a 41 per cent lower heart-attack risk than teetotallers, although the effect wasn't so great for women of the same age. And scientists from the Karolinska

Institute in Sweden found that women who drank the equivalent alcohol to half a glass of wine a day had a lower risk of heart attacks. (The other thing that they found helped reduce heart attacks was eating a lot of fruit and vegetables, and it's possible that there may be some kind of combination effect, where the compounds in the fruit, vegetables and alcohol work together. And the people were also eating healthy diets in general – so eating a dreadful diet and just adding a half a glass of wine won't work!)

It appears that *any* alcohol helps a little, but red wine appears to have the most beneficial effect. This is due to antioxidants and polyphenols, which have a protective effect on the blood vessels. Which, of course, is also beneficial to brain function.

One unit of alcohol is equivalent to:

- Half a pint of average-strength beer, lager or cider (3–4% alcohol by volume)
- Small glass of wine (9% alcohol by volume)
- Standard pub measure (25ml) of spirits (40% alcohol by volume)
- Standard pub measure (50ml) of fortified wine, e.g. sherry, port (20% alcohol by volume)

Remember that a lot of pubs and restaurants serve wine in large 175ml (two-unit) glasses, and many people are used to drinking pints of beer or lager, and doubles. Also, 'home measures' are also notoriously generous.

SUPPLEMENTS

Even if you're eating a really healthy diet, it's difficult to get enough of some of the nutrients that are vital for brain health from your food, and in these cases we would recommend taking a supplement.

This is particularly important in the case of the omega essential fatty acids. Also, recent research has shown that many people need to take vitamins C and B complex together with zinc and magnesium for the omegas to be processed in the body into the useable form. Although I am very much in favour of omega-3 supplementation and firmly believe every child and adult in the country should be taking a daily dose, yet again without a diet free from additives and the right exercises it will only serve its one essential function, which may be better than nothing, but is simply not enough if you have specific problems.

The essential omegas

It is virtually impossible, even with the healthiest diet, to get enough of the essential fatty acids that are so important to the brain.

The official daily recommended intake of EPA and DHA together is 500mg for adults (the equivalent of a generous portion of an oily fish such as salmon twice a week), but this is the recommendation for *heart* health, and the brain is likely to be wanting significantly more. For this reason, the dosage for people with learning disorders would be expected to be higher.

To give you an idea of how difficult we find it to get enough of our essential omegas EPA and DHA, the average intake in the UK is a mere 100 to 150mg per day.

It's probably safe to say that if you suffer from the kind of problems discussed in this book, your essential fatty acid stores will be severely run down. The guideline amounts of approximately 500mg per day are only intended for 'general good health and maintenance', and the Tinsley House Clinic recommends doubling the normal dose for the first three months of supplementation, in order to top up your stores of these vital fats.

I recommend a product called Efalex, which provides a combination of omega-3 and omega-6 nutrients including DHA, EPA and AA. It is suitable for children aged two and over and adults, and is available from Boots, health food stores, chemists or supermarkets. For further information see www.efalex.co.uk.

Which supplement?
Here's what to look for:

- Enough of the essential fatty acids.
- Purity – poor-quality fish-oil supplement may be contaminated with heavy-metal pollutants such as mercury.
- Packaging – EFAs are sensitive to heat and light, so they should be packaged in dark-coloured containers, and not

stored in full sunlight. Capsules are less vulnerable to heat and light degradation than liquid oils.

● Buy fish oil, and not fish *liver* oil (as in cod liver oil). Liver, including fish liver, is extremely high in vitamin A. In order to get sufficient EPA and DHA from fish liver oil, you could consume dangerously high levels of vitamin A.

Omega-3 and -6 supplements are available in various forms but beware, some of these products, notably those directed at children, contain colorants and aspartame, which would seem to make no sense at all.

VEGETARIAN ALTERNATIVES

The only 'ready-made' sources of the omega-3 EFAs EPA and DHA – the forms actually used by the brain – are the oils in fish and seafood. However, in theory the body *can* convert another EFA, found in flaxseeds and their oil, into EPA and DHA. In practice, though, this conversion is slow and inefficient, especially in people suffering from learning disabilities and other developmental delay syndromes. This means that, unless you are a strict vegetarian, fish oils are superior to flaxseed oil supplements. You can also buy vegetarian EPA and DHA supplements sourced from micro-algae.

Zinc

The other supplement recommended by the Tinsley House Clinic is zinc. Zinc deficiency (and also magnesium deficiency) is one of the nutrient deficiencies most commonly seen in children with developmental delay syndrome (especially those with ADHD symptoms), and a similar deficiency can be expected in adults suffering from learning disabilities.

Because of this observed link between zinc deficiency and ADHD symptoms, scientists have carried out carefully monitored clinical trials to test whether zinc supplements could help ADHD children.

In a study of 44 children by scientists in Iran, the children receiving the medication methylphenidate along with 55mg zinc sulphate (the equivalent to 15mg elemental zinc) showed a greater improvement in their symptoms than those on methylphenidate and a dummy pill with no active ingredient.

Another double-blind study, this time in Turkey, backs up the Iranian research. Four hundred children suffering from ADHD were given either 150mg zinc sulphate supplements (more than in the Iranian study) or dummy pills. After twelve weeks, the zinc group were less hyperactive and impulsive, and were better at socialising with others. This effect was particularly strong in the older children with low levels of zinc and essential fatty acids, perhaps suggesting that zinc might be as effective, or even more so, in adults with similar symptoms.

Both of these were randomised and double-blind studies – the most reliable kind of research. Neither the children and their parents, nor the people who distributed the 'real' zinc and the dummy supplements, knew who was receiving the real treatment – the only people who knew were the scientists behind the trial. This removed the possibility of bias (if parents and children expected to see certain results, or if the people handing out the pills unconsciously revealed hints as to whether they were getting 'real' or dummy treatment).

Most zinc supplements available in the UK provide zinc in quantities up to 15mg, but the studies on zinc sulphate used supplements containing up to 55mg zinc. However, it is not possible to suggest dosages for individual patients without knowing their nutritional status, and being able to monitor their reaction to the treatment. For this reason I recommend that you speak to your doctor if you feel that zinc sulphate could help you.

Other supplements

If you've not been eating healthily for some time, your reserves of some nutrients may be run down, and for this reason it may be a good idea to take a good-quality multivitamin/multimineral. You don't need a 'megadose' – just look for one that gives you 100 per cent of the recommended amount.

But don't think this gives you an excuse to continue eating unhealthily – a supplement is just a safety net, a backup to top you up, rather than a substitute for a balanced diet.

The Supplement Regimen

- Essential fatty acids: a double dose for three months and the normal dose (300–500mg EPA + DHA) thereafter
- Zinc sulphate: 15mg (adults only)
- Magnesium: 100% of daily recommended amount
- Vitamin C: 100% of daily recommended amount
- Vitamin B complex: 100% of daily recommended amount

The UK recommended intake for magnesium is set at 300mg for men and 270mg for women.

In the USA the figure has recently been revised upwards and it is now recommended that the intake should be 400mg per day for men aged 19 to 30 and 420 for those over 30; the figures for women under and over 30 are 300mg and 310mg per day respectively.

The UK/USA recommended intake for zinc is 15mg for children over 12 years and male adults and 12mg for female adults.

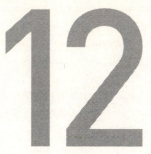

OTHER BRAIN-RELATED DISORDERS

Now that you know the huge impact your diet has on your brain, its function and your mental health, you can see how eating a healthy diet could reduce your risk of suffering from other brain-related conditions.

DEPRESSION

Depression is the most common mental disorder in the UK, accounting for a huge amount of suffering, not to mention economic performance and lost working days. Although depression is a very real medical condition (it's not just 'the blues'), there is a lot you can do, diet-wise, to reduce your risk of suffering from it, and even supporting or aiding recovery.

Population studies show that countries where large amounts of fish are eaten suffer less from depression than non-fish-eating countries – and this links in with the brain's requirement for the omega-3 EFAs found in fish, especially oily fish. Clinical trials have also found omega-3s to be helpful in treating depression, though the doses used were high (up to 9.6g EPA+DHA per day). If you suffer from clinical depression, you should be receiving care from a doctor, and discuss any supplements with him or her before taking them.

Several studies have found that people experienced low mood when they were low in vitamin B1 (thiamine), and their mood improved when they improved their levels of the vitamin. Good sources include lean pork, liver and unrefined grains.

Selenium is also important to the brain, and research has found a link between low levels and depression. One study found that the depression improved after five weeks of selenium supplementation. Good dietary sources include lean meat, fish, eggs, nuts (especially Brazils) and seeds.

Low folate levels also appear to be linked with low mood and depression, emphasising the need to maintain your level of this B vitamin, found especially in green leafy vegetables.

ALZHEIMER'S, OTHER DEMENTIAS AND AGE-RELATED MENTAL DECLINE

It's unsurprising that there is a link between omega-3 EFAs and Alzheimer's, dementia and the gradual mental decline associated with old age (Alzheimer's is a kind of dementia, but not all 'dementias' and forms of age-related mental decline are due to Alzheimer's). Several large-scale population studies have found links between fish (especially oily fish) consumption and protection against these conditions. Other studies found a connection between high intakes of saturated fats and dementias. There certainly seems to be a link between high cholesterol levels and Alzheimer's, so doing the things that lower your cholesterol must surely help:

- Minimise saturated fat
- Eat moderate amounts of unsaturated fats
- Eat foods containing soluble fibre such as oats
- Take exercise

Keeping a check on your salt intake could also reduce your risk of dementia, since salt can raise your blood pressure, increasing the risk of the 'mini strokes' that can lead to so-called vascular dementia – which basically means problems in the brain caused by circulation problems.

Vegetarians also appear to be at lesser risk of Alzheimer's than meat eaters, though the reason is unclear. It's likely that a high intake of fruit and vegetables, beans and pulses is a factor, though low levels of saturated fats (found in high amounts in many animal products) could also contribute.

Antioxidants are one reason for the protection offered by fruit and vegetables – these nutrients mop up the harmful free-radical molecules that damage blood vessels and contribute to dementias. One population-based study found that 500mg of vitamin C and 400iu vitamin E (both antioxidant vitamins) daily were linked to a lower risk of Alzheimer's.

Another study found that people who ate at least three servings of vegetables per day slowed their rate of cognitive (mental) decline by roughly 40 per cent compared with those who ate less than one helping per day – a decrease equivalent to about five years of younger age. Interestingly, fruit failed to produce the same protective effect, though it is still rich in nutrients, low in calories, and should definitely be part of a healthy diet. Especially since another study suggests that compounds found in apples help prevent age-related mental decline.

An amino acid (protein building block) found in the blood, called homocysteine, could also play a role in deterioration of the brain – high homocysteine levels are associated with increased Alzheimer's risk. You can help to lower your homocysteine levels by eating a diet rich in EFAs, wholegrains, and antioxidant-rich foods such as fruit, vegetables, nuts and seeds.

Interesting but early-stage research suggests that the curry spice turmeric could also slow the rate of mental decline and help prevent Alzheimer's. The protective effect is thought to be due to a compound called curcumin.

Keep your brain sharp – the Mediterranean way

If you want to reduce your rate of age-related mental decline, the 'Mediterranean diet' seems a good place to start. This way of eating, long associated with healthy hearts, involves low-fat protein mainly from fish and poultry, beans and other pulses, nuts and seeds, large amounts of fruit and vegetables, and moderate amounts of unsaturated oils, mainly olive oil.

Two recent studies found a link between improved mental skills in the elderly and eating fish. The more fish eaten, the greater the benefit, especially for the oily fish that are rich in essential fatty acids.

EXERCISE – GENERAL AND SPECIFIC

GENERAL EXERCISE

If you want to be healthy, it's not enough just to eat healthily, you have to be active too.

If you haven't been in the habit of taking regular physical exercise for a while it is perhaps a good idea to have some indication of your current fitness level before starting, and you should consult your GP before starting any exercise programme if you are overweight, a smoker, or suffer from any chronic health conditions such as heart problems, type-2 diabetes or arthritis.

One simple way to gain an insight into your current health status is to calculate your body mass index (BMI). Doctors use the body mass index as a way to assess whether or not a patient needs to lose weight. The simple calculation is based on comparing a person's weight with their body height and it applies equally well to men and women.

Body mass index (BMI) is a measure of body fat based on your height and weight that is used to measure whether adults are the 'correct' weight. There are admittedly problems with BMI – it isn't accurate for children, the elderly or heavily muscled people such as bodybuilders and conditioned athletes – but it is a good guide-line as to whether an average person is the correct weight.

To calculate your body mass index divide your weight in kilograms by the square of your height in metres using a calculator, or if you are on the internet simply type in 'Calculate Body Mass Index' to a search engine and follow the instructions.

- Underweight = BMI less than 18.5
- Normal weight = BMI 18.5–24.9
- Overweight = BMI 25–29.9
- Obese = BMI 30–39.9
- Severely obese = BMI 40 or greater

The good old days

The machine age, the age of technology or the IT era, whatever you want to call it, has brought forth amazing advantages in taking the drudgery out of many of the mundane tasks we all need to perform each day, but it has also taken with it the exercise associated with those tasks. No longer do you need to scrub the washing or push the lawn-mower up and down with sweat dripping from your brow, and although you probably eat less in a day than previous generations, this lack of exercise that was built into daily chores can pile on the pounds unless you take positive action via your diet and add some form of leisure pursuit or sporting activity to your weekly schedule.

Apart from the fact that my parent's generation did not have such things as washing machines that would wash, spin and dry at the touch of a button or an array of power tools for every job that needs doing, they also didn't have colour televisions, DVD players, computers or any of the other electronic gadgets to amuse themselves – or the time to be a world-class couch potato. Aside from the more physical nature of both work and home life, parents and grandparents would most likely have followed more active leisure pursuits, simply because the more idle pastimes of today were not available. To get some idea of how much time you spend on sedentary (sitting on your bottom) activities, total up the number of hours you spend watching the TV, surfing the internet, playing computer games or using an electronic game.

Many families today have two or more cars, which means that no one has to walk to the bus stop to go to work or walk to the local shops to get a loaf of bread. More and more local shops are disappearing,

COULD IT BE YOU?

which necessitates taking the car to the nearest supermarket for the weekly shop. The advent of fridges, freezers, chill cabinets and food processing has changed the way we shop, where we shop and what we buy. It is the ability to chill, freeze or process that has made the super-market possible and, because we too can store quantities of food safely in our own fridges and freezers, we don't have to shop on a daily basis. This is all very well but insidiously along the line we have changed not only where we shop but, more importantly, what we buy.

Moving food around the world, manufacturing food in bulk and providing a shelf life means modern foods generally have to be treated chemically or have chemicals added to them (or be frozen). In order that you can have what you want when you want, be it in season or not, a huge transport system must be in place, generating a massive carbon footprint. However, I believe it is bulk manufacturing and the processes involved in this to ensure the look, taste and shelf life of our food that are the real problem, and the reason why you now eat 8 to 9lb (4kg) of chemicals a year.

Labour-saving gadgets, tools and machines are not just found in the home. They have been part of the workplace since the Industrial Revolution, but now virtually every occupation has its own labour-saving devices, be it the power screwdriver or nail gun used by the carpenter or the computer now found in every office in the land. This has not only reduced the amount of physical work that needs to be done in any one day, but it has also taken away many of the fine, skilled movements that were part and parcel of many occupations and activities – print setting or technical drawing, for instance – which can now be done by computer aided technology.

Therefore, apart from needing to give serious thought to what we are eating and the impact this may have upon your health, it is also very necessary to put a little physical activity back into the work-place, the home and your leisure time. We tend to think about exer-cise simply in terms of muscular activity, but it is not just your muscles that benefit from a little extra gardening or a workout at the gym.

THERE IS MORE TO EXERCISE THAN MEETS THE EYE

- Helps to control weight and prevent weight gain
- Builds and tones muscles, including the heart

- Reduces the risks of osteoporosis later in life
- Lowers cholesterol
- Reduces the risk of stroke, heart and arterial disease
- Reduces the risk of diseases such as cancer and type-2 diabetes
- Supports the immune system, keeping you well
- Builds a healthy appetite
- Helps you sleep well
- Relieves stress
- Improves co-ordination
- Boosts self-esteem – the feel-good factor

FIT AS A FIDDLE

So what do you need to do to be truly fit? Ideally we all need a well-rounded blend of exercise that should include:

- Aerobic fitness – to build endurance and strengthen our heart and lungs
- Strength – to increase or maintain muscle mass
- Flexibility – to improve suppleness and balance
- Weight-bearing exercise – for strong healthy bones

Aerobic exercise

Aerobic exercise is any physical activity that exercises the heart and lungs (the cardiovascular system) – gets the heart pumping and works up a bit of a sweat. Although this may conjure up images of Lycra-clad bodies doing step exercises or whatever else is the current craze, it doesn't necessarily have to involve leotards and posing.

It could include:

- Power walking
- Running
- Cycling
- Swimming
- Team games, such as football or netball
- Tennis and badminton
- Ice skating
- Dancing
- Judo

Strength exercise

Strength exercise, usually referred to as weight training, doesn't just mean lifting weights down at the gym. Strength exercise is any activity that helps to build and strengthen the muscles that move and support the body. This could include such things as sit-ups, press-ups or even attending a ballet class, which requires a considerable amount of body strength if performed well. Resistance bands come in various strengths and can provide a very user-friendly form of exercise for the older, less active person.

Flexibility exercise

Most sports and active games naturally require degrees of flexibility, but so do everyday activities like stretching up to reach a top shelf, or bending down to pick up the debris left behind by the children. If you feel that you are not very flexible or you are getting on in years, you might want to consider joining a yoga class or trying Tai Chi, a gentle martial arts form that is excellent for developing flexibility, poise and balance.

Weight-bearing exercise

At least twice a week you should take part in some form of activity that will help build bone or help maintain bone density – so-called 'weight-bearing exercise'. Any form of exercise that involves standing up and moving about counts as weight bearing.

Good examples are:

- Walking
- Running
- Skipping
- Tennis
- Football
- Netball
- Hockey
- Trampolining

Keep it in the family

If you have children, show them that you think exercise is important by being active yourself. Make fitness a family affair – every one of you needs exercise, and research has shown that parents who enjoy physical activity themselves are more likely to encourage their children to be active. Try to plan at least one family activity each week – it doesn't need to be expensive or even cost anything at all.

Why not try:

- A hike in the country
- A climb up a local hill
- A visit to a playground
- A game of badminton in the garden
- A game of cricket or football in the park
- A walk along a river or a trip to the beach (beach games in winter are great fun and the sands are less crowded)
- A long bike ride
- Flying a kite
- A visit to an ice rink
- A trip to the local swimming pool
- Family 'orienteering' – in other words, a walk/jog following a map

A walk in the park

Remember, there are plenty of ways to boost activity levels, without doing actual exercise, by incorporating more general activity into your daily life.

- Walk to the shops if at all possible
- If you have children walk to school, if it's not too far
- Use the stairs rather than a lift or escalator wherever possible
- Walk the dog (if you have one) twice a day
- Be as active as possible in the garden
- Make love often

SPECIFIC EXERCISES FOR DEVELOPMENTAL DELAY SYNDROME

A testing time

Before attempting these specific exercises it is essential to carry out the series of simple tests that follow in order to establish which side of the body – and hence the brain – needs to be exercised. You will need a friend or partner to complete the tests. Following each test tick the appropriate box – Left or Right.

TEST 1

Stand in front of a friend or your partner with your feet together, hands by your side and eyes closed. Have them gently but firmly tap your upper arm just below shoulder level, firstly on the left and then on the right. Have them repeat this two or three times. Have them note if you lose balance, move a foot or an arm. Tick the box for the side that you fell towards or the opposite side to the foot or arm that moved. That is, if the right arm or foot moves you tick the *left* box.

TEST 2

Sit in front of your partner with your arms outstretched and the index finger of each hand pointing directly at their nose. With your eyes closed you must touch your nose and then point at their nose, firstly with the index finger of the right hand and then with the left. This should be repeated several times consecutively and must be done with the eyes closed. Have them note if one finger repeatedly misses the nose or if there is a slight hesitation before the finger touches the nose. Tick the box for the finger that repeatedly misses the target or has a slight tremor before making contact.

TEST 3

Sit in front of your partner and stretch your arms out in front of you. With your eyes open, turn your hands to the palm-up position and rapidly alternate the movement: palms down/palms up. Have your partner look for the hand that goes out of sync first or the elbow that bends and then tick the appropriate box.

TEST 4

Sit facing your partner, with your elbows by your side and forearms outstretched in front of you, palms upwards. Then turn your hands palm down/up as rapidly as possible while keeping your elbows by your side. Have your partner note which hand goes out of sync first or which wrist bends producing a waving movement. Tick the box as to left or right.

TEST BOX

	RIGHT	**LEFT**
TEST 1	☐	☐
TEST 2	☐	☐
TEST 3	☐	☐
TEST 4	☐	☐
TOTAL	☐	☐

Now look at your Test Box above. If three or more ticks are left or right (in other words, the tests show a majority for *either* left or right) you are safe to proceed with the following exercises. If you are unsure about any of the results or the results are evenly mixed you should consult an experienced practitioner.

The following exercises should only be started once you have completed the tests above and you are confident of the results. Here we will assume that you have ticked three or four of the **LEFT** boxes. If you have ticked 3 or 4 of the **RIGHT** boxes then simply swap right for left in the instructions given below.

The following exercises should be carried out daily along with the progressive stair-walking exercises we introduced in Chapter 9 (which are repeated here for convenience). You must do Exercise 1 daily, plus at least one of the other two.

Progressive Stair-walking Exercises

1. With hands by your sides, head in the neutral position and eyes closed, walk up and then down three stairs, three times, three times a day. **Never go higher than three stairs.** When you can do three repetitions perfectly, do five, then seven, then ten.

2. Once you have mastered forward stair-walking, do it backwards with the same progressions.

3. Once you can stair-walk forwards and backwards, start forward stair-walking again, but this time carrying a tray with a plastic tumbler full of water on it.

Daily Lateral Exercises

1) Twice a day, when cleaning your teeth – use your left hand and stand on your left leg.

2) Teach yourself to use a yo-yo using your left hand. Learn as many tricks as possible.

3) Stand on your left leg while listening to a piece of music. Conduct the orchestra with your left hand only and sing along to the music if possible. (Best done in private!)

Once you have been doing exercises 1 and 2 for a couple of weeks you can then listen to music at the same time. The music should be listened to via the **LEFT** ear only and should not be accompanied by any singing. You will need to use an earplug-type earphone to achieve this.

Once you have been doing these activities for around six weeks, do the four tests again and see if you and/or your partner see an improvement.

The physical exercises should be continued until they are perfected. If you continue to struggle with the exercises or show no sign of progress after, say, two months, consider contacting a Tinsley House Treatment Centre for advice – www.tinsleyhouseclinic.com 'Find a clinic' is on the home page.

So how does it work?

The general exercises for the brain's cerebellum are designed to challenge the cerebellum, making the 'weaker' side come up to speed.

LEFT/RIGHT specific cerebellar exercises are designed to challenge one cerebellar hemisphere (side of the brain) via the need to balance and/or produce unaccustomed movements.

LEFT/RIGHT specific brain exercises are designed to challenge known functions of the left/right cerebral hemispheres. To give you an example of this, look at the letter T below:

```
I I I I I I I I I I I I
I I I I I I I I I I I I
        I I I
        I I I
        I I I
        I I I
        I I I
```

If you look at the letter 'T' from a distance you are using the right side of the brain. Once you look at the detail and see it is made up from the letter 'I' you are using the left side of the brain. The right side of the brain sees the big picture while the left side examines the detail. There are a great many functions which are specifically left or right and some which can be attributed to specific areas of the brain on one side. By knowing the sidedness of these functions it is possible to 'exercise' set areas of the brain.

Later, when describing how the various computer programs work, we will look at not only specific areas of the brain but also the types of neurons within pathways of the brain within these specific areas that can be activated by known stimuli – sights, sounds, etc. Therefore, by knowing the certain colours, pattern sizes and frequency of change that are necessary to stimulate certain neurons, one area of the brain can be activated; as these areas of the brain do not work in isolation, then areas at the back of the brain, for instance, can be made to activate areas of the prefrontal cortex (another part of the brain).

GETTING MORE HELP

Once the diet and supplements are in place and the exercises are progressing well you are going to need a little help from a health professional if you feel that further treatment is necessary. For instance, if your primary problem is with reading speed and you suspect you may have secondary dyslexia, then you will need to have certain tests carried out in a clinic or optometrist's office that has the facility to carry out this kind of testing before you can start the computer-generated treatment plan. Unfortunately, all the computer-generated treatment programmes have to be prescribed to fit the specific needs of the individual or dispensed by an optometrist and cannot be simply purchased at a computer store. We will consider the use and provision of these computer-generated programmes more fully in the next chapter.

The exercises and activities described above are intended to help children/adults with learning/behavioural problems. If you have any concerns about your health you should contact a health professional for advice.

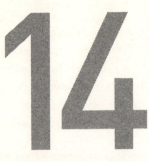

COMPUTER-GENERATED TREATMENTS

Computers, or rather computer software, have over the years been developed to help with the diagnosis of a variety of conditions. In terms of learning and behavioural disabilities they have proven to be an invaluable tool. The tests described below are available at Tinsley House Treatment Centres (THTC) throughout the UK and at the few centres currently operating abroad. Some of the assessments will also be available elsewhere, so it might be worthwhile asking your nearest optometrist if they have the facilities to carry out such tests.

As they are treatment programs and not games they have to be provided in accordance with the individual requirements of the law of the country in which they are prescribed, and are therefore not available at computer-software outlets. Many also have authorisation codes built into them so their use can be strictly controlled and monitored, thereby ensuring that only the person that has been given the program uses it.

THE DIAGNOSTIC TOOLKIT

The physiological blind-spot imager

The place where the optic nerve exits the back of the eye is called the optic disc, and because it does not have light-detecting photoreceptor cells it cannot 'see'. For this reason it is called the physiological blind spot. However, as the two eyes are not perfectly aligned (in parallel), each eye can fill in for the other eye so that (usually) our field of vision is complete, with no actual blind spot.

Try this little test

Hold the book up very close in front of you. Cover your RIGHT eye and keep your LEFT eye on the letter X below. Now slowly move the book away from you, still focusing on the X. The O will disappear as it passes over the blind spot while the A remains still visible.

A   O   X

The physiological blind-spot imager uses this simple fact in a very clever way. The person being tested rests their chin and forehead against a special frame, which is positioned at a set distance in front of a computer screen. An eye patch is placed over one eye while the person being tested is asked to focus on a target in the centre of the screen. As the test begins a cursor moves off towards the edge of the screen and the person being tested has to say when the cursor first disappears and then reappears. The cursor then moves back into the established blind spot and then moves out in eight different directions while the person being tested says when the cursor reappears. The eye patch is then placed over the other eye and the procedure is repeated.

Now comes the clever bit. The computer then produces two images of the blind spot, together with a measurement of the area each covers. These images often vary considerably in size, which of course the actual blind spot could not do unless it was very swollen (a condition called papilloedema) and this would be picked up during a routine examination of the eye. The difference in the size of the blind spot images is due to variations in the processing speed of each hemisphere of the brain and the time taken for the person to register and say 'Yes'. It therefore provides a very good assessment as to how the individual brain hemispheres are functioning as a whole.

The visual therapy assessment (VTA)

This very accurate assessment of how well the eyes function while in convergence was the brainchild of Dr Jeffrey Cooper and Rod Bortel in the USA. The program provides slow-moving (pursuits) and fast-moving (saccades) targets, which the person being tested – seated sixteen inches in front of the screen – has to follow. To ensure they continue to do this, they have to indicate by hitting the up/down/right/left buttons on the keyboard depending on which way the target is pointing. It then generates random dot stereograms – 3D pictures – which cause the eyes to move into convergence (together) or divergence (apart) or jump between the two. The range of convergence/divergence that the person can see is measured by the program in fractions of units called dioptres. It also tests for correct alignment of the eyes and the ability to accommodate in convergence.

This test is used to provide an objective assessment following the sometimes-subjective manual test using an isopter (inverted cocktail stirrer). Not only does it provide a very accurate assessment of the patient's ability to move their eyes before starting treatment, it also provides an objective assessment as to how the treatment is progressing and when the treatment can be terminated.

The perceptual therapy assessment (PTA)

Although the perceptual therapy system (PTS) was primarily designed by Sidney Groffman to help children with learning disabilities, it works equally well with adults. The PTS test consists of three separate tests: for visual closure (the ability to recognise a picture that is gradually forming), visual span (the ability to remember a sequence of letters shown on the screen) and the tachistoscope, which flashes letters or numbers up on the screen for a fraction of a second. At the end of the test the computer prints off the test results. A PTA demonstration can also be performed in the clinic as an assessment of the person's ability to complete the various parts of the program. As we will see later, both the PTS and HTS treatment programs can be modified to suit the patient's particular needs or ability.

The Visagraph

The Visagraph is the culmination of over seventy years of eye-movement recording and reading research and is an objective measurement tool for reading efficiency (fluency). The examiner places the Visagraph goggles on the subject's head and adjusts them in relation to the pupils of the eyes. The subject then reads a short selection from a test booklet that is reading-age related and answers questions to determine how well he or she has understood. Infrared sensors in the goggles record the patient's eye movements while he or she silently reads the appropriate text. Eye-movement characteristics are then automatically analysed by the computer software and detailed reports that provide insight as to 'how' the individual reads are then generated.

Apart from again providing a very accurate objective measurement of eye movements beforehand, the program can also be used to monitor progress once the treatment programme has been put in place. More than that, it allows the subject being tested to see how their eyes move when they are reading by superimposing a cursor that represents the eye movement (tracking) over the top of the text the subject has just read. Apart from producing stacks of figures and graphs that allow progress to be followed accurately, this ability for the subject to see for themselves the reduction in fixations (when the eyes stop tracking) or regressions (when the eyes move right to left) is very rewarding and proof of the progress being made.

On the basis of the Visagraph assessment, computer-generated treatment programmes can be put in place that the subjects can either download from the internet or load onto their computer from a CD. The subject then completes a set number of treatment sessions in the comfort of their own home, while their progress can be monitored by the subject's practitioner via an internet link. Many of the programs used have this facility, which means the patient doesn't have to make so many visits to the prescribing practitioner's surgery or office, and makes it possible to treat anyone, anywhere.

THE WORKS

The home therapy system (HTS)

HTS is the treatment of choice for anyone with secondary dyslexia or with dyslexia as a main symptom of their developmental delay. If you think you may have secondary dyslexia (accommodation/convergence failure) try this simple test:

Convergence test

Have someone sit in front of you and bring a pencil with an eraser on the end in towards your nose from about eighteen inches (45cm). Try to keep your eyes fixed on the eraser. Have your partner bring the pencil in towards your nose and back again at least three times. Your partner should look at the bridge of your nose and note if both your eyes move in towards your nose as the pencil approaches and move smoothly out as it moves away. If one eye is slow to move in or moves in but then fails to hold convergence, you should consider having a VTA test carried out at a Tinsley House Clinic or by an optometrist.

If your problem is purely secondary dyslexia then a full assessment for aspects of developmental delay may not be necessary and you can use the HTS program at home while being monitored via the internet by your practitioner. However, if you suspect there may be more to it than just secondary dyslexia, that is, you have other prominent symptoms, then a full assessment by an experienced practitioner is essential.

The beauty of the HTS program is that it is used at home, so you don't have to make regular visits to a treatment centre. It will auto-load onto your computer and once installed provides an instruction video which shows you exactly what you will need to do, plus the opportunity to practise each part of the exercise before you actually run the program. It is a smart program in that it monitors your progress each day and as you achieve set targets it will automatically take each individual part of the program up to a different level. Once you have attained the level of proficiency required in each section, that part of the program is dropped, which reduces the amount of time it takes to complete the exercises each day. This process of dropping parts of the program will continue until all the sections have been completed successfully, when the program will tell you to contact your eye doctor.

If you have access to the internet your performance review (scores achieved) will be automatically uploaded to the HTS directory in the USA from where your practitioner can access your file. Having monitored your progress over the weeks your practitioner can now remotely switch your program from automatic to manual mode and, based on your performance, tell you which parts of the program need a little extra work. This facility also means that if you are struggling with a part of the program, your practitioner can send you a message of encouragement or modify the program to make things easier for you. At some point, usually six to eight weeks after starting to use the program and again towards the end of the treatment, it is necessary for you to retake the VTA test, which means a trip to the clinic or optometrist's office.

Once the HTS program is completed I personally like to carry out a Visagraph assessment as well as a VTA assessment to ensure that the eyes are tracking as they should be now that convergence is functioning normally. If there is still a problem this can be easily remedied by using another home-based computer-generated treatment programme, either Reading Plus® or ADR.

Perceptual therapy system (PTS)

Secondary dyslexia is due to poor convergence/accommodation, but although degrees of convergence failure are present in over 50 per cent of the subjects tested in a clinic, some people require help as well with other aspects of visual processing within the brain itself. In this situation (and this usually goes hand in hand with other prominent symptoms of developmental delay) the use of the perceptual therapy system is required. This program has all the same very useful features in that it auto-loads, uploads to a directory in the USA and can be monitored remotely – but it has the advantage of addressing issues other than the mechanics of vision.

If you have problems with phonics (sounds), differentiating left from right, reversal of words or letters such as 'b' for 'd', if you have been diagnosed as having dyslexia or attention deficit, if you are or have underachieved academically or have difficulties remembering things, this could be the best treatment for you.

While the HTS programs train you to focus – converge your eyes and fixate on a target – the PTS program goes still further and *helps* you to focus. It helps you to concentrate on what you are doing, and learn. Although the program has a game-like nature, each individual part of the program has a sound theoretical basis and causes perceptual learning to take place effortlessly. The PTS program provides a daily training session that lasts about twenty minutes and addresses such things as hand-eye co-ordination, attention span and the various components of visual processing and learning.

Hemistim II

The Hemistim program was the brainchild of a colleague of mine in Holland called Roland Blaauw, who designed a computer program that can be configured to produce moving patterns that will selectively stimulate one of two kinds of cells in the brain that are involved in vision. That in itself is pretty amazing, but the real benefit of using this program is that it is also known which areas of the brain the two types of cell talk to, so by changing the configuration the level of stimulation to these areas can be adjusted to suit the individual needs of the subject. As the stimulation needs to be presented to just one side of the brain, during the treatment session the subject sits to one side of the computer and looks at a book placed to the right (usually) or left of the screen. I use *Where's Wally* or 'wordsearch' books, as the act of searching provides an added bonus to the treatment.

Tracking and reading fluency

In terms of reading and understanding what you read, the final stage of treatment involves improving reading fluency. To achieve this we use one of two computer-generated treatment programmes. Once the first, called Reading Plus®, has been prescribed it is downloaded from the internet and monitored by your practitioner over a period of months. It is a very comprehensive treatment plan that comes from the Visagraph people and therefore has a great deal of research behind it. However, it is not cheap and this may prove to be a problem for people on a low income, particularly when you take into consideration other fees you may have already incurred to get you to this point in your treatment.

The ADR Dynamic Reading Program has the considerable advantage of being much cheaper than the Reading Plus® system, so it's very affordable to anyone who needs treatment and comes with the back-up of a very friendly helpline team at HTS.

Reading Plus®

Reading Plus® courses are designed to address important visual and perceptual skills that allow you to focus your energies on reading to learn rather than just struggling to read. Most of us assume that effective reading develops automatically as we learn to read aloud, but unfortunately this is not typically the case.

As we have seen, in order to read effectively we must firstly be able to bring the eyes into convergence and then be able to track (move across the page smoothly). Reading-behaviour habits will emerge that will either help or hinder our effectiveness in reading for the rest of our lives. These skills involve our ability to co-ordinate our eyes, track along lines of text, and quickly and accurately recognise and store words in our short-term memory. These basic skills are unconscious and cannot be controlled, but we can develop them with proper training.

ADR Dynamic Reading Program

This is another excellent program from the VTA/HTS/PTS people in America. The program follows three simple progressions designed to make reading a naturally more fluent process by reducing the number of 'stops' and right-to-left eye movements.

Moving Text Dynamic Reading

In Moving Text Dynamic Reading, the material to be read remains in the centre of the screen and does not move down the page from top to bottom; this means that fast eye movements are not required. This prevents you from losing your place and your concentration when the print moves down to the next line. This step introduces the concept of 'Dynamic Reading', which emphasises fluency, and improvement in the eyes' ability to track across the page, or move from left to right.

Standard Dynamic Reading

In Standard Dynamic Reading, the print moves left to right and top to bottom. This step continues the emphasis on fluency, and improvement in the eyes' ability to track across the page, or move from left to right. It also introduces the added complexity of top-to-bottom reading.

Whole Line Dynamic Reading

In Whole Line Dynamic Reading, the material to be read does not move left to right but is presented as an entire line at a time. The patient must generate their own left-to-right eye movements while processing the information. The reading material moves down the page one line at a time to the end of the passage. The speed is determined by the patient's reading rate and level of understanding. This is a critical bridge to normal reading.

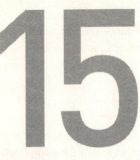

THE BRAIN-FRIENDLY EATING PLAN

Eating a balanced diet that's high in 'brain-friendly nutrients' can help support any treatment for learning or behaviour disorders. It's also the kind of diet to help anyone fulfil their full potential – both in terms of brain function and general health.

The kind of diet we recommend contains low-fat protein, moderate amounts of healthy fats, wholegrain starchy carbohydrates and plenty of fruit and vegetables. It's based around simple, home-cooked meals, using fresh ingredients, rather than relying on processed foods and ready-meals. It doesn't involve spending hours in the kitchen, and you're even allowed treats and desserts!

Here is a sample seven-day eating plan, with all the recipes you need to follow it. You should also make sure that you drink at least 1.5 litres of water per day (about 8–10 good sized glasses).

THE SEVEN-DAY PLAN

SUNDAY
Breakfast:
Poached egg and grilled tomato on a toasted wholemeal English muffin. A low-fat fruit yogurt and a small glass of pure fruit juice.

Snack:
Two rye crispbreads lightly spread with low-fat cream cheese.

Lunch:
Roast lamb studded with garlic and rosemary, roast potatoes, carrots, Brussels sprouts and parsnips. **Dutch apple crumble** with a scoop of good-quality vanilla ice cream.

Snack:
A pear. A small glass of semi skimmed milk.

Supper:
Homemade French bread ham, mushroom and pineapple pizza with salad. A mango and raspberry fruit salad, topped with two tablespoons of low-fat fromage frais and a drizzle of honey, if needed.

Roast lamb studded with garlic and rosemary
Serves 4

1 lamb leg joint
4 cloves of garlic, cut into slivers
A few small sprigs of rosemary

1. Preheat the oven to 180°C/Gas 4.
2. Using the sharp point of a knife, make a series of slits on the surface of the joint. Insert slivers of garlic and small sprigs of rosemary into the slits to flavour the meat during cooking.
3. Roast the joint for the time required for the size of the joint.

Dutch apple crumble
Serves 4

450g/1lb cooking apples, peeled, cored and sliced
50g/2oz sultanas
25g/1oz light, soft brown sugar
½tsp cinnamon
150ml/¼pint water
For the crumble:
50g/2oz olive-oil spread (suitable for baking)
100g/4oz plain flour
75g/3oz light, soft brown sugar
25g/1oz oats
25g/1oz walnuts, chopped

1. Preheat the oven to 200°C/Gas 6.
2. To make the crumble, rub the olive spread into the flour until the mixture resembles fine breadcrumbs. Stir in the sugar, oats and walnuts.
3. Place the sliced apple and sultanas in an ovenproof dish, sprinkle over the sugar and cinnamon and mix together. Pour over the water. Microwave on high for 1½–2 minutes to slightly soften the fruit.
4. Spoon the crumble mixture over the fruit and press down lightly. Bake in the oven for 45 minutes until the crumble is lightly golden and the apples are soft.

Homemade French bread ham, mushroom and pineapple pizza

Serves 4

1 thick wholemeal French stick loaf (at least 40cm/16 inches long)
1 small can chopped tomatoes
1 tbsp tomato puree
¼tsp dried Italian seasoning or mixed herbs
100g/4oz mushrooms, thinly sliced
3 slices of lean, cooked ham, diced
6 slices pineapple, tinned in juice not syrup, drained and quartered
4tbsp mature Cheddar cheese, grated

1. Preheat the oven to 180°C/Gas 4.
2. Cut two 20cm/8 inch lengths from the French stick. Cut each length in half lengthways to produce 4 bases for your pizzas.
3. Place the chopped tomatoes, tomato puree and herbs into a saucepan and boil gently for 10 minutes to produce a thick sauce. Allow to cool and spread over the cut sides of the bread slices.
4. Top with the mushroom slices, diced ham and quartered pineapple slices. Sprinkle over the cheese. Bake in the oven for 12–15 minutes until the cheese has melted and the bread is crisp. Serve with a large salad.

MONDAY
Breakfast:
Two medium eggs, scrambled, on a slice of wholemeal toast. A chopped pear topped with ½ carton of low-fat natural yogurt and a drizzle of honey (optional).

Snack:
A **mini rock bun** and handful of grapes.

Lunch:
A chicken salad – slices of chicken with lettuce, watercress, cucumber, spring onions, halved cherry tomatoes and a fat-free vinaigrette or a teaspoon of low-fat mayonnaise. (If you need to take your lunch to work in a plastic container, take the dressing separately so that the salad does not go limp and soggy.)

Snack:
A peach or pear and a small glass of pure fruit juice or semi-skimmed milk.

Dinner:
Grilled mustard topped salmon fillet with steamed/boiled new potatoes, mange tout, sweetcorn and two grilled tomato halves. A **baked eating apple stuffed with chopped dates** and served with two tablespoons of low-fat natural fromage frais.

Mini rock buns
Makes 20

200g/7oz wholemeal self-raising flour
100g/4oz white self-raising flour
¼tsp mixed spice
100g/4oz olive-oil spread (suitable for baking)
175g/6oz sultanas
50g/2oz ready-to-eat dried apricots, finely chopped
75g/3oz light, soft brown sugar
1 medium egg, lightly beaten
125ml milk

1. Preheat the oven to 200°C/Gas 6.
2. Place the wholemeal flour, white flour and mixed spice into a mixing bowl. Rub in the olive spread. Stir in the sultanas, finely chopped apricots and the soft brown sugar. Stir in the beaten egg and add the milk a little at a time until you have a moist but firm 'rocky' mixture.

3. Drop dessertspoonfuls of the mixture onto a baking sheet lined with non-stick baking parchment. Leave 5cm between each of the buns to allow them to spread slightly during cooking.
4. Bake for 15 minutes or until the buns are firm and brown. Do not overcook. Allow to cool and store in an airtight container.

Grilled mustard topped salmon
Serves 4

4 salmon fillets
3tbsp grainy mustard
1tsp olive oil

1. Place the salmon on a sheet of foil on a grill pan. Brush with the olive oil and spread the mustard over the fillets.
2. Place under the grill for 4–6 minutes or until the fish is cooked through. Take care not to overcook or the salmon will dry out. Serve the salmon on a bed of watercress.

Baked apple stuffed with chopped dates*
Serves 4

4 large eating apples
12 dates, finely chopped
Juice of 2 oranges

1. Preheat the oven to 180°C/Gas 4.
2. With the tip of a knife score through the skin around the centre of each apple. Remove the cores of the apples using an apple corer.
3. Place the chopped dates in a small bowl and add a small quantity of the orange juice. Mix together and use to fill the centre of each apple.
4. Place the apples in an ovenproof dish and pour over the remaining orange juice. Cover the dish with a piece of kitchen foil. Bake in the oven for 30–40 minutes or until the apples are tender.

*As a change from dates try stuffing apples with sultanas or raisins.

TUESDAY

Breakfast:

A bowl of porridge, made with semi-skimmed milk and topped with a small handful of raspberries. A slice of wholemeal toast, lightly spread with olive-oil spread and a low-sugar jam.

Snack:

4 ready-to-eat unsulphured dried apricots and a dessertspoon of sunflower seeds.

Lunch:

A portion of **healthy hummus** or 100g cottage cheese with pineapple, with 4 rye crispbreads and a selection of vegetable sticks – carrots, celery, red pepper and cucumber. Two plums or a kiwi fruit.

Snack:

An apple and a digestive biscuit. A small glass of semi-skimmed milk.

Dinner:

A **grilled minted lamb chop** with mashed potatoes, carrots, cabbage or baby spinach. Two grilled pineapple rings with two tablespoons of low-fat natural fromage frais.

Healthy hummus

Makes 6 portions

1 large can of chick peas, drained and rinsed
1 small clove garlic, roughly chopped
1tbsp olive oil
1tbsp lemon juice
3tbsp low-fat natural yogurt
Salt and freshly ground black pepper

1. Place all of the ingredients, except the salt and pepper, in a blender and whiz until smooth. Taste and adjust the seasoning by adding a little salt and pepper if needed. Cover and chill in the fridge.

Grilled minted lamb chops
Serves 4

4 lamb chops (or leg steaks), fat removed
2tbsp mint jelly
1tsp water
2tsp vinegar

1. Combine the mint jelly and water in a small china ramekin and place in the microwave on high for 20 seconds to melt the mint jelly. Stir in the vinegar.
2. Brush both sides of the chops with the mint mixture and grill the meat until it is cooked to your liking. Serve with mashed potatoes and seasonal vegetables.

WEDNESDAY
Breakfast:
Two slices of wholemeal bread topped with mushrooms (sautéed in a little water) and 4 grilled tomato halves. A banana.

Snack:
A **wholemeal sultana scone** lightly spread with low-sugar jam, if liked.

Lunch:
A tuna and salad sandwich. (If you buy a sandwich ensure that it is wholemeal bread and contains low-fat dressing). A low-fat fruit yogurt and a handful of grapes.

Snack:
A finger of **homemade fruity bar** and a small glass of semi-skimmed milk.

Dinner:
Cajun chicken with roasted vegetables, homemade potato wedges and a green salad. Three stewed plums topped with two tablespoons of low-fat natural fromage frais and two tablespoons of no-sugar no-salt muesli.

Wholemeal fruit scones
Makes 12–14 scones

225g/8oz wholemeal self-raising flour
1tsp baking powder
50g/2oz butter
25g/1oz caster sugar
50g/2oz sultanas
150ml/¼ pint milk
Milk, to brush tops

1. Preheat the oven to 230°C/Gas 8 and place a non-stick baking tray into the oven.
2. Sieve the flower and baking powder into a mixing bowl and rub in the butter until the mixture resembles fine breadcrumbs. Stir in the sugar and the sultanas. Add sufficient milk to make a soft dough.
3. Lightly flour a pastry board or clean work surface and turn out the dough. Knead very lightly to form a ball. Pat or roll out to about 2.5cm/1 inch thick and cut into rounds using a 6cm/2½ inch round cutter.
4. Remove the hot baking tray from the oven and place the scones onto it. Brush the tops of the scones with milk and return the baking tray to the oven quickly.
5. Bake for 8–10 minutes until the scones are well risen and golden. Do not overcook or they will be dry. Cool on a wire rack.

Cajun chicken with roasted vegetables
Serves 4

1 red onion, peeled and cut into wedges
1 large courgette, cut into thick slices
12 mushrooms, halved
1 red pepper, deseeded and cut into large chunks
1 green or yellow pepper, deseeded and cut into large chunks
8 cherry tomatoes
2tbsp olive oil
1tsp Cajun seasoning
4 chicken breasts, skin removed

1. Place the onion wedges in a saucepan and cover with boiling water. Place on the heat and gently simmer for 3 minutes. Drain.
2. Place the prepared courgette, mushrooms, pepper, tomatoes and drained onion wedges into a large bowl, add 1tbsp of olive oil and sprinkle over half of the Cajun seasoning. Toss lightly to coat the vegetables with oil and spice. Transfer to a large non stick baking tray.
3. Brush the chicken breasts with the remaining olive oil and sprinkle over the remaining Cajun seasoning. Add to the vegetables in the baking tray.
4. Bake in the oven for 25–30 minutes or until the chicken is cooked through. Serve with a salad and a small jacket potato.

Homemade potato wedges

4 large potatoes, washed but not peeled
1tbsp olive oil
Ground black pepper, Cajun spice, paprika or chilli powder

1. Preheat the oven to 200°C/ Gas 6.
2. Boil the unpeeled potatoes whole for 10 minutes. Drain and cool under cold water. Cut the potatoes in half lengthways, then cut each half lengthways again. Cut each of the quarters into thick wedges. Dry on kitchen towel.
3. Put the oil into a large bowl and add the potatoes. Toss the wedges to lightly coat in the oil.
4. Lay the wedges on a non-stick baking tray (or non-stick baking paper). Sprinkle lightly with one of the spices. Put the wedges into the oven and bake for 25–35 minutes or until the potatoes are tender. Turn them a couple of times while they are cooking so that they brown evenly.

THURSDAY
Breakfast:
A 2-egg mushroom omelette with a grilled tomato. A slice of wholemeal toast spread with olive-oil spread and a little honey, Marmite or low-sugar jam. A banana.

Snack:
A yogurt pot filled with plain popcorn tossed in a pinch of paprika or teaspoon of grated Parmesan cheese.

Lunch:
An egg and cress wholemeal baguette, accompanied by 4 cherry tomatoes. A low-fat fruit yogurt.

Snack:
A mini rock bun (see Monday's recipe) and a small glass of semi-skimmed milk.

Dinner:
Speedy spaghetti Bolognese with a **tomato, onion and mint salad. A raspberry and yogurt 'Crannachan'.**

Speedy spaghetti Bolognese:
Serves 4

450g/1lb lean minced beef
1 medium onion, chopped
1 large can chopped tomatoes
2tbsp tomato puree
100ml/3½ fl oz vegetable stock or water
100g/4oz mushrooms, sliced
1½tsp Italian seasoning
2 bay leaves
Salt and freshly ground black pepper
1tbsp Worcestershire sauce
6 black olives, stoned and halved (optional)
225g/8oz spaghetti
4tsp Parmesan cheese, finely grated

1. Place the minced beef in a large non-stick saucepan and fry gently, stirring to break up the meat, until the mince has browned. Drain off any fat which has come out of the meat. Add the onion and continue cooking for 3 minutes. Stir in the chopped tomatoes, tomato puree, stock or water, mushrooms, Italian seasoning and bay leaves. Add the Worcestershire sauce and olives, if you are using them. Bring to the boil, reduce the heat, cover the pan

and simmer for 25–30 minutes until the sauce has thickened slightly. Season to taste with salt and freshly ground black pepper. (If the sauce is not thick enough simmer uncovered for a further 5 minutes.)

2. Cook the spaghetti in plenty of boiling water according to the packet instructions, drain and serve. Place the spaghetti into serving bowls and top with the Bolognese sauce and a sprinkling of Parmesan cheese.

Tomato, onion and mint salad
Serves 4

2tbsp olive oil
1tbsp vinegar
½tsp honey
Freshly ground black pepper
4 large tomatoes
1 medium onion
2tsp fresh mint, chopped

1. Combine the olive oil, vinegar, honey and freshly ground black pepper in a small bowl.
2. Slice the tomatoes into rings and arrange on a plate. Peel and thinly slice the onion and arrange over the tomato slices. Sprinkle over the mint and drizzle over the dressing.

Raspberry and yogurt 'Crannachan'
Serves 4

200g/7oz raspberries
300g/10½oz low-fat natural yogurt
4tsp honey
6 oatcakes, lightly crushed
3tbsp chopped walnuts
8 mint leaves to decorate

1. Take 4 sundae glasses or small thick tumblers. Rinse the raspberries in cold water and place on a pad of kitchen towel to absorb any water. Reserve 8 raspberries for decoration.

2. Using half of the raspberries, place them in the base of each glass, top with a layer of yogurt and a drizzle of honey. Add a layer of crushed oatcake followed by the remainder of the raspberries. Complete with a layer of yogurt and a drizzle of honey. Top with the chopped nuts and decorate with two raspberries and two mint leaves.

FRIDAY
Breakfast:
A hard boiled egg and a slice of lean, unsmoked ham with two slices of wholemeal bread lightly spread with olive-oil spread. A banana.

Snack:
A **fruity snack square.**

Lunch:
A chicken and salad wholemeal sandwich with a low-fat dressing. A carton of fresh fruit in juice and a low-fat fromage frais.

Snack:
An apple or an orange and 2 oatcakes. A small glass of semi-skimmed milk.

Dinner:
Baked haddock 'rarebit' with boiled or steamed new potatoes, broccoli, asparagus or mange tout. Two homemade **Scotch pancakes** with ½ a banana cut into circles and 2tbsp low-fat natural fromage frais. Add a drizzle of honey if desired.

Fruity snack squares
Makes 16

3tbsp runny honey
75g/3oz olive-oil spread (suitable for baking)
50g/2oz light soft brown sugar
100g/4oz sultanas or seedless raisins
50g/2oz ready-to-eat unsulphured dried apricots, finely chopped
60g/2½oz ready-to-eat prunes, finely chopped
50g/2oz walnuts or pecans, chopped

2tbsp milk
175g/6oz porridge oats
½tsp mixed spice
50g/2oz seeds (any combination of pumpkin, sesame, sunflower)

1. Preheat the oven to 190°C/Gas 5 and lightly grease an 18cm × 18cm square baking tin.
2. Place the honey, olive-oil spread and sugar in a saucepan and cook over a gentle heat for 5 minutes, stirring all the time, until it resembles a thick sauce. Add all the remaining ingredients and mix together well.
3. Transfer the mixture into a greased baking tin and bake in the middle of the oven for 25–30 minutes until golden brown and firm. Remove from the oven. Allow to cool in the tin for 10 minutes then mark into small squares. Leave in the tin to cool completely before cutting along the marks. Store in an airtight container.

Baked haddock 'rarebit'
Serves 4

4 haddock fillets, skin removed
Olive oil for brushing
2tsp mild mustard, Dijon or German
3 medium tomatoes, sliced
4tbsp mature Cheddar cheese, grated

1. Preheat the oven to 180°C/Gas 4.
2. Place the haddock fillets on a non-stick baking tray and lightly brush with olive oil. Spread a little mustard over the top of each fillet. Arrange the tomato slices on the top and sprinkle with the grated cheese.
3. Bake the fillets in the oven for 15–18 minutes or until the fish is cooked. The cooking time will depend on the thickness of the fish.

Scotch Pancakes
Makes 12

100g/4oz wholemeal self-raising flour
2tsp sugar
Pinch of salt

1 egg, beaten
150ml/¼pint milk

1. Place the flour into a mixing bowl with the sugar and pinch of salt. Make a well in the centre and add the beaten egg. Beat well, gradually incorporating the milk until you have a smooth batter.
2. Heat a heavy based non-stick frying pan or flat griddle and wipe with a little oil on a piece of kitchen towel. Drop tablespoons of the pancake mix onto the hot pan, well spaced apart. Cook for 2 minutes until bubbles rise to the surface. Gently turn them over and cook for a further minute.

For a change add a tablespoon of sultanas and a squeeze of lemon juice to your pancake mix, or stir in a tablespoon of fresh blueberries or raspberries.

SATURDAY

Breakfast:
A slice of wholemeal cheese on toast with grilled tomatoes. A low-fat natural yogurt topped with a handful of blueberries and a drizzle of honey, if needed.

Snack:
A **fruity snack square** (see Friday's recipe) and an apple.

Lunch:
Homemade vegetable and lentil soup (or a portion of fresh soup from a 'healthy range' from the chiller cabinet at the supermarket) with a warmed crusty baguette.

Snack:
A banana.

Dinner:
Honey and orange chicken with **garlic and chilli baked baby jacket potatoes,** green beans and broccoli. **Plum and almond crunch** with a scoop of good quality vanilla ice cream.

Homemade vegetable and lentil soup
Serves 4

1.2 litres/2 pints vegetable or chicken stock
175g/6oz dried red lentils
4 rashers of bacon, all fat removed and diced
1 onion, diced
1 large carrot, diced
1 medium potato, peeled and diced
1tsp chopped parsley
Salt and freshly ground pepper

1. Place the stock, lentils, bacon, onions, carrots and potato into a large saucepan and simmer for 50 minutes. Add the parsley, season to taste and simmer for a further 10 minutes.
2. Remove the saucepan from the heat and using a slotted spoon remove 3 spoonfuls of vegetables and set aside in a bowl. Liquidise the remaining soup in a blender until smooth. Return to the pan and add the vegetables you had set aside. Serve piping hot with homemade wholemeal bread croutons and a crispy wholemeal roll.

Wholemeal bread croutons
Remove the crusts from 4 thick slices of wholemeal bread and cut into small squares. Arrange the squares of bread on a non-stick baking tray or sheet of baking parchment and lightly spray with low-fat olive oil spray. Bake in a low oven (150°C/Gas 2) until the croutons are crisp. Shake the tray a couple of times while they are cooking.

Honey and orange baked chicken
Serves 4

1tbsp runny honey
1tbsp olive oil
2tbsp mild mustard, Dijon or German
Finely grated rind of an orange
Juice of ½ orange
½ orange, cut into wedges
4 chicken breasts, skins removed
Freshly ground black pepper

1. Preheat the oven to 200°C/Gas 6.
2. Place the honey, olive oil, mustard, orange rind, juice and wedges into a shallow dish and mix together. Add the chicken breasts and spoon over the marinade.
3. Transfer to a non-stick baking tray and pour over any remaining marinade. Cover with foil and bake for 20 minutes, then remove the foil and cook for a further 5 minutes. Check that the chicken is cooked – the juices will run clear when you stick a knife into the thickest part of the breast. If the juices are not clear continue cooking for a further 5 minutes or until the chicken is cooked through. Serve with garlic and chilli baby baked potatoes, green beans and broccoli.

Garlic and chilli baby jacket potatoes

Serves 4

600g walnut-sized new potatoes, scrubbed but not peeled
2tbsp vegetable oil
1 medium red onion, peeled and finely chopped
2 cloves garlic, crushed
¼tsp dried crushed chillies (optional)
300ml/1 pint vegetable stock
Freshly ground black pepper
3tbsp parsley, chopped

1. Peel a thin strip around the centre of each potato – to prevent the skins splitting when the potatoes are cooking.
2. Place the oil in a large non-stick frying pan and gently sauté the onion, garlic and chilli until they are softened.
3. Add the stock, freshly ground pepper and chopped parsley. Tip the potatoes into the pan and arrange them in a single layer. Partially cover the pan with foil or a lid – so that steam can escape – and simmer for 12–15 minutes until the potatoes are tender. Transfer the potatoes to a serving dish and pour over the remaining sauce.

Plum and almond crunch
Serves 4

450g/1lb sweet red plums
25g/1oz Demerara sugar
To make the crunch:
50g/2oz butter
175g/6oz wholemeal plain flour
75g/3oz caster sugar
25g/1oz porridge oats
50g/2oz slivered almonds

1. Preheat the oven to 180°C/Gas 4.
2. Cut the plums in half and remove the stones. Place the plums cut side down in a shallow ovenproof dish. Sprinkle over the Demerara sugar.
3. Melt the butter in a small saucepan over a low heat so that it does not burn.
4. Place the flour, caster sugar, oats and almonds into a bowl and add the melted butter. Mix together to form a rough mixture. Sprinkle over the plums in an even layer. Bake in the oven for 25–30 minutes until the crunch is golden.

IN SUMMARY

I hope you have found this book to be both interesting and informative. While every attempt has been made to present the information in a way that is easily understood and the self-help elements were designed to be as user-friendly as possible, if you are unsure about anything or feel that you require further help, you should contact an experienced practitioner for further advice.

The team at the Tinsley House Treatment Centres may be contacted via: www.tinsleyhouseclinic.co.uk

GLOSSARY

Accommodation/convergence failure – the inability of the eyes to move in towards the nose when looking at something close up e.g. when reading.

Acetylcholine – a substance used by nerves to send messages to other nerves.

Afferentating – causing messages to be sent into the nervous system.

Allo – the **allocortex** is a part of the cerebral cortex (outer layer of the brain) characterised by having fewer cell layers (3) than the isocortex (6).

Alpha-linolenic acid – an omega-6 essential fatty acid.

Amino acids – the 'building blocks' that make up proteins.

Anterior cingulate – the anterior cingulate cortex (ACC) is the frontal part of the cingulate cortex, which resembles a 'collar' around the corpus callosum (the body that joins the two cerebral hemispheres).

Antioxidants – chemical components of foods that neutralise harmful free radical molecules that damage the body's cells.

Apoptosis – the name given to the programmed cell death that occurs during development of the brain. Cells that do not migrate or do not make contact with other neurons die.

Arachidonic acid – a polyunsaturated fatty acid that is essential for growth.

Archiocortex – the outer layer of the brain is called the cortex. There are three types of cortex – archio, paleo and neocortex. The first two are called primitive cortex (older) while the last type is the newest in terms of brain evolution.

Artificial sweeteners – artificially produced chemicals, many times sweeter than sugar, added to food for sweetness.

Aspartame (also known as E951) – the best known (and most infamous) artificial sweetener, alleged to contribute to a variety of health problems.

Asperger's syndrome – a disorder in which the individual shows marked deficiencies in social skills, does not like change, often has obsessive routines and becomes preoccupied with particular subjects.

Attention deficit disorder (ADD) – an inability to focus/concentrate on the job in hand, with a tendency to be easily distracted. Tends to go hand in hand with ADHD – it is a classic symptom of developmental delay.

Attention deficit hyperactivity disorder (ADHD) – as for ADD above but with aspects of hyperactivity and impulsivity.

Autism (true) – affects about 1 in 5,000 children, being four times more common in boys than girls. It has been thought for some time to be due to abnormal brain development and now would appear to be due to a lack of spindle cells (VEN). Autistic children avoid eye contact, shun affection, do not understand other people's emotions/feelings, have problems making friends and cannot adjust to the rules of society.

Autistic spectrum disorder (ASD) – affects 9 in 1,000 children. These children display autistic tendencies and it may well prove to be an extreme form of developmental delay due to reduced numbers of spindle cells (VEN) or greatly impaired spindle cell development.

Azo dye – a synthetic dye, usually red, brown or yellow, which makes up about half the dyes we use.

Benzoate – chemical used as a food preserver.

Blood sugar level – the amount of sugar in the blood stream at any one given moment of time.

Bpoptosis – a term coined in 2005 by R Pauc to cover the period of time during which the second wave/generation of human brain cells develop, migrate and make contact with other neurons.

Brainstem – the part of the nervous system that joins the brain to the spinal cord: it contains many of the vital centres – vital because without them you die.

Caffeine – stimulant chemical, found in coffee and also tea, chocolate, energy drinks and some cold remedies.

Calories – unit of measurement for the energy found in food.

Carbohydrates – a component of food, used to produce energy in the body. Can be divided into sugary carbohydrates and starchy carbohydrates.

Carcinogen – a substance thought to cause cancer.

Central Nervous System (CNS) – the brain, brainstem and spinal cord.

Cerebellar hemisphere – the cerebellum has a middle section (vermis = worm) with a large lobe on either side called a hemisphere.

Cerebellum – literally 'little brain' that lives in the very back of the skull under the brain.

Cerebral hemisphere – the name given to either side of the brain.

Cholesterol (HDL) – the 'good' kind of cholesterol that reduces your risk of clogged arteries, heart disease and stroke.

Cholesterol (LDL) – the 'bad' kind of cholesterol that increases your risk of clogged arteries, heart disease and stroke.

Choline – a dietary component of many foods. Forms part of many major phospholipids.

Chromosomal – to do with chromosomes, which are the threadlike structures found in the nucleus of cells and which carry the genes.

Comorbidity – when two or more conditions appear together at the same time.

Compliance – obeying the rules.

Congenital – present at birth.

Convergence failure – the inability to bring the eyes in towards the nose, necessary for close vision.

Corpus callosum – the body of white matter joining the two cerebral hemispheres.

Cranial Nerves – 12 pairs of nerves found at the base of the brain and brainstem.

Cross Cord Reflexes – messages that get passed from one side of the spinal cord to the other so that we can do things like walking, swimming etc.

Developmental Delay Syndrome (DDS) – a slowing in the development/maturation of the brain which causes the symptoms of dyslexia, dyspraxia, attention deficit, hyperactivity, obsessions and tics to occur.

Diabetes – usually refers to diabetes mellitus, a disorder characterised by excessive urinary excretion. Common types are Type 1 diabetes, Type 2 diabetes and Gestational – occurring during pregnancy.

Diaschisis – put simply this is when one area of the brain does not work too well because an area it normally communicates with has a problem. So it is a bit like a couple having a row and not talking to each other.

Disaccharide – A sugar made up of two 'sugar units' joined together. Examples include sucrose (table sugar) and lactose (the sugar found in milk).

Docosahexaenoic Acid – an omega-3 essential fatty acid.

Dopamine signalling – messages sent from one nerve to another using a special substance, a neurotransmitter called dopamine.

Dressing dyspraxia – difficulty dressing.

Dysarthia – inability to produce clear speech.

Dysdiadochokinesia – the inability to make rapidly alternating movements e.g. turning the hands palm up/down.

Dyslexia – a term used to cover a variety of learning difficulties.

Dysmetria – inaccurate movements.

Dyspraxia – an inability to perform learned movements accurately: can take many forms and has been found to be present in association with the other symptoms of developmental delay in over 90 per cent of children.

Echolalia – repeating what you have just heard.

Eicosanoids – signalling molecules, derived from omega-3 and omega-6 essential fatty acids, involved in immunity and inflammation.

Eicosapentaenoic acid – an omega-3 essential fatty acid.

Empty calories – food/calories that provide energy (and can lead to weight gain) with little or no other nutritional benefit. A label often applied to sugar!

Emulsifier – a substance that helps to keep together substances that normally would not go together e.g. oil and water.

Equasym – Equasym tablets and Equasym XL capsules both contain the active ingredient methylphenidate hydrochloride, which is a type of medicine called a stimulant. It is used to treat attention deficit hyperactivity disorder (ADHD) in children.

Fat emulsifier – a substance that helps to keep together substances that normally would not go together e.g. oil and water.

Fibre – the indigestible component of food. Can be divided into soluble fibre, which helps you maintain healthy cholesterol levels and is therefore good for heart health, and insoluble fibre, which is good for your digestive system.

Flavour/flavoured (on labels) – foods labelled 'flavour' (e.g. 'strawberry flavour') need not contain any of the real ingredient (in this case, strawberries) – their taste can come entirely from artificial additives. Foods labelled 'flavoured' (e.g. 'strawberry flavoured') must actually contain that ingredient.

Foetal Alcohol Spectrum Disorder – a fairly recent new term to cover both the physical and neurological effects to the foetus due to the maternal ingestion of alcohol during pregnancy.

Foetal distress – when the foetal heartbeat rises or drops dramatically.

Folic acid – a member of the B vitamin group, needed by pregnant women to reduce the risk of neural tube defects (such as spina bifida). Could also benefit heart health.

Functional dominance – when one area of the brain is superior or dominant in function.

Functional foods – foods which claim to have health benefits beyond normal nutrition. Many have had their nutritional properties artificially boosted, for example by the addition of 'friendly bacteria', or omega-3 essential fatty acids.

Gamma-linoleic acid – an omega-6 essential fatty acid.

Ghrelin – a hormone, produced by the stomach before meals, which stimulates appetite.

Gigantopyramidal cells – very large motor neurons found in the mid cingulate gyrus (inside wall of the brain).

Glue ear – a condition when the middle ear is filled with a gluelike fluid instead of air.

Glycaemic Index (GI) – a measure of the amount that a food increases blood sugar level.

Glycaemic Load (GL) – a more sophisticated form of the Glycaemic Index, that takes into consideration the amount *per serving* that a food increases blood sugar level.

Hormones – a chemical messenger transported around the body in the bloodstream.

HUFAs – highly unsaturated fatty acids.

Humectant – a substance that attracts water and therefore helps to keep a food substance moist.

Hydrogenated fats – fats that have been artificially altered to change their hardness and increase their keeping properties. Found in many manufactured foods, they form a large proportion of the harmful 'trans' fats in our diets.

Hygroscopic – readily absorbs water.

Hypothalamus – a tiny area of the brain weighing c. 4 grams that controls basic functions such as hunger, thirst, oxygen levels in the blood, etc.

Inositol – a food substance found notably in cereals.

Interconversion – the conversion of one essential fatty acid to another form.

Interneurons – small nerves that interconnect with other nerves.

Irritable Bowel Syndrome (IBS) – a multi-faceted disorder thought to be due to a disturbance in the interaction between the intestines, the brain and the autonomic nervous system, which alters the regulation of bowel function. It is characterised by abdominal pain or discomfort and is associated with a change in bowel pattern, such as loose or more frequent bowel movements, diarrhoea and/or constipation.

Lecithin – a fat-like substance called a phospholipid which is a fat emulsifier.

Linoleic acid – an omega-6 essential fatty acid.

Meconium – the first stool a baby passes.

Methylphenidate Hydrochloride – a central nervous system stimulant better known as Ritalin.

Monosaccharide – a single unit sugar, for example glucose or fructose.

Monosodium Glutamate (MSG) – a flavour enhancer, also known as E621. Implicated in behavioural symptoms such as hyperactivity.

Monounsaturated fat – a 'healthy' kind of fat that benefits your cholesterol levels. Olive oil, and also the oils found in nuts and seeds, are good sources.

Motor planning – how the brain plans what it is it wants to do.

Motor skills – the ability to carry out physical things you have learned to do.

Myelin – the fatty insulation that covers nerve fibres.

Myelination – the process that takes place during development when certain nerves are wrapped in myelin.

Myopic – being nearsighted.

Neocortex – in terms of evolution, the newest parts of the brain.

Neuroanatomy – the anatomy of the nervous system.

Neuroepithelium – specialised tissue in the developing brain that produces firstly neurons and then all other brain cells.

Neurologist – an expert in neurology.

Neurology – the study of the nervous system.

Neurons – cells found in the brain, brainstem, spinal cord and nerves.

Neurotoxic – brain poisoning.

Neurotransmitter – a chemical substance that passes messages from one neuron to the next.

Nystagmus – the flickering of the eyes from side to side.

Obsessive-compulsive disorder (OCD) – is characterised by a recurrent urge to carry out ritualistic behaviour patterns: it is a common symptom of developmental delay – to a certain extent we all have minor aspects of compulsive behaviour, only becoming a problem when it occurs to such a degree that it takes over a person's waking life.

Omega-3 and -6 fatty acids – forms of polyunsaturated essential fatty acids (polyunsaturates) that are particularly important for brain development and function. They are also beneficial for heart health. The best food sources are oily fish, but they are also found in flaxseeds and other nuts and seeds.

Oppositional Defiance Disorder – European description: conduct seen in children below ten years of age characterised by markedly defiant, disobedient or provocative behaviour. American description: a pattern of hostile, negative, defiant behaviour lasting at least six months, during which four of the following occur: often loses temper, often argues with adults, often actively defies or refuses to comply with requests/rules, often deliberately annoys others, often blames others for his/her mistakes, is easily annoyed, is often angry, is often spiteful.

Otoacoustic Emission Tests – a hearing test of inner ear function.

Otoscope – the device used by doctors for looking in the ear.

Paleocortex – one of the more primitive (older) types of the outer layer of the brain (cortex).

Partially hydrogenated fats – similar to hydrogenated fats (see glossary entry), and another important dietary source of harmful 'trans' fats.

Peripheral nerves – nerves that leave the spinal cord.

Peripheral nervous system – the nervous system is divided in the central nervous system – brain/brainstem/spinal cord – and the peripheral nervous system – all the nerves that leave or enter the spinal cord.

Peripheral testing – the testing of the nerves that leave the spinal cord to supply the arms and legs principally.

Phosphatidyl serine – a component of the cell membrane called a phospholipids.

Phosphoglyceride – a type of phospholipids.

Phospholipid – a fatty component of the cell wall.

Phytochemical – literally 'plant chemicals'. Beneficial nutrients found in plant-based foods such as fruit, vegetables, nuts and seeds.

Polysaccharide – a chain made up of individual sugar units.

Prebiotic – non-digestible compounds added to foods and food supplements, to 'feed' the beneficial 'friendly bacteria' in the human gut.

Prefrontal cortex – a large area of brain (in humans) at the front of each cerebral hemisphere.

Probiotic – the beneficial 'friendly bacteria' that inhabit the gut.

Prosody – the musical quality of language, as opposed to a flat monotone.

Prostaglandins – a member of a group of fats made from omega-3 and -6.

Protein – a nutrient, needed for body growth, maintenance and repair.

Psychometric tests – tests to measure brain function.

PUFA – polyunsaturated fatty acid.

Ritalin – a trade name for Methylphenidate Hydrochloride, a central nervous system stimulant used in the 'treatment' of ADHD.

Saturated fat – a class of fat, usually solid at room temperature, found mainly in animal products such as meat, eggs and dairy products. Has the effect of raising the level of 'bad' LDL cholesterol.

Savant ability – an extraordinary skill/ability e.g. the ability to remember pages of telephone numbers or the ability to say on which day a person's birthday will fall in any given year.

Schizophrenia – mental illness characterized by impairments in the perception or expression of reality, most commonly manifesting as auditory hallucinations (hearing voices), paranoid or bizarre delusions (false beliefs) or disorganized speech and thinking.

Sensory integration – the blending of sensory input into the body so that it becomes meaningful.

Sequestrant – a food additive that binds with metals, which might have got into the food by accident, thus making them inert.

Serotonin – a neurotransmitter believed to play an important role in the regulation of mood, sleep, vomiting, sexuality and appetite.

Sodium chloride – common table salt.

Spindle cells (von Economo cells) – special brain cells (neurons) that develop four months after birth in humans: they are only found in the brains of the great apes, whales and Man. It is considered that these cells and the development of the prefrontal cortex (the front of the brain) is what make us truly human.

Statemented – the 1993 Education Act (UK) provided a code of practice giving guidance on how to identify and assess the special educational needs (SEN) of children: if it is felt that a child has SEN, then a formal request can be made to have the child statemented, which if formally accepted will ensure that the child's needs are met.

Synaesthesia – a condition in which sensory experiences are misinterpreted in the brain so that the sufferer may taste words or feel colours.

Synaptogenesis – the forming of synapses (gaps) between neurons across which chemical messages can pass.

Syndrome – a collection of signs and symptoms that appear together.

Temporal sequencing – fitting events into a time frame.

Titubation – rocking to and fro.

Tourette's syndrome – is a class of tic disorder.

Trans fats – a class of fats with similar negative health effects to saturated fats. Hydrogenated and partially hydrogenated fats and oils are their main source in the diet, but they are also naturally found in smaller amounts in animal products.

Tympanometry tests – special hearing tests which assess how well the ear-drum and middle ear is functioning.

Vagal brake – one way in which the brain controls the heart rate, blood pressure and respiration rate.

Ventouse – an assisted birth using suction to pull the baby through the birth canal.

von Economo neurons – see Spindle cells

Wholegrains – unrefined cereal grains, such as those found in wholemeal bread, brown pasta, wholemeal noodles, as well as brown rice, buckwheat, millet and oats.

INDEX